# [ mindfulness in motion ]

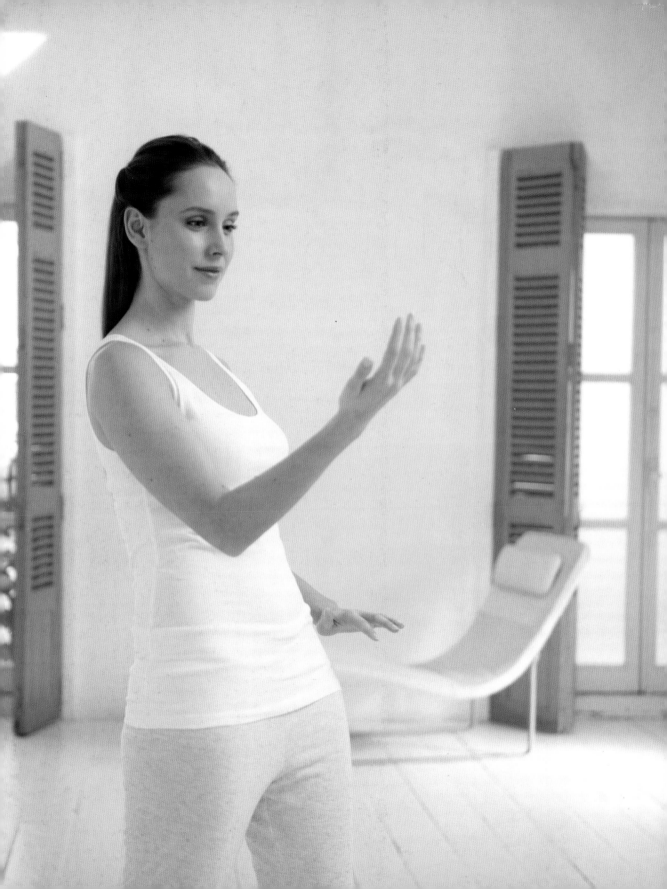

# mindfulness
# in motion

## a happier, healthier life through
## body-centred meditation

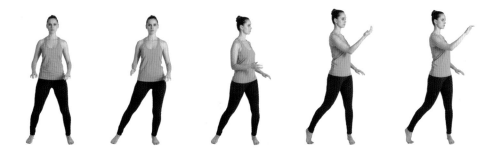

### Dr Tamara Russell

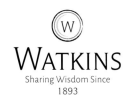

WATKINS
Sharing Wisdom Since
1893

**Mindfulness in Motion**
Dr Tamara Russell

First published in the UK and USA in 2015 by
Watkins, an imprint of Watkins Media Limited
19 Cecil Court
London, WC2N 4EZ

enquiries@watkinspublishing.co.uk

Managing Editor: Sandra Rigby
Development Editor: Fiona Robertson
Design: Blok Graphic
Picture Research: Jennifer Veall
Production: Uzma Taj
Commissioned Photography: John Englefield

A CIP record for this book is available from the British Library

ISBN: 978-1-78028-581-8

10 9 8 7 6 5 4 3 2 1

Typeset in Gentona
Colour reproduction by XY Digital, UK
Printed in China

**Publisher's note**: The information in this book is not intended as a
substitute for professional medical advice and treatment. If you are
pregnant or are suffering from any medical conditions or health
problems, it is recommended that you consult a medical professional
before following any of the advice or practice suggested in this book.
Watkins Media Limited, or any other persons who have been involved in
working on this publication, cannot accept responsibility for any injuries
or damage incurred as a result of following the information, exercises or
therapeutic techniques contained in this book.

**www.watkinspublishing.com**

# contents

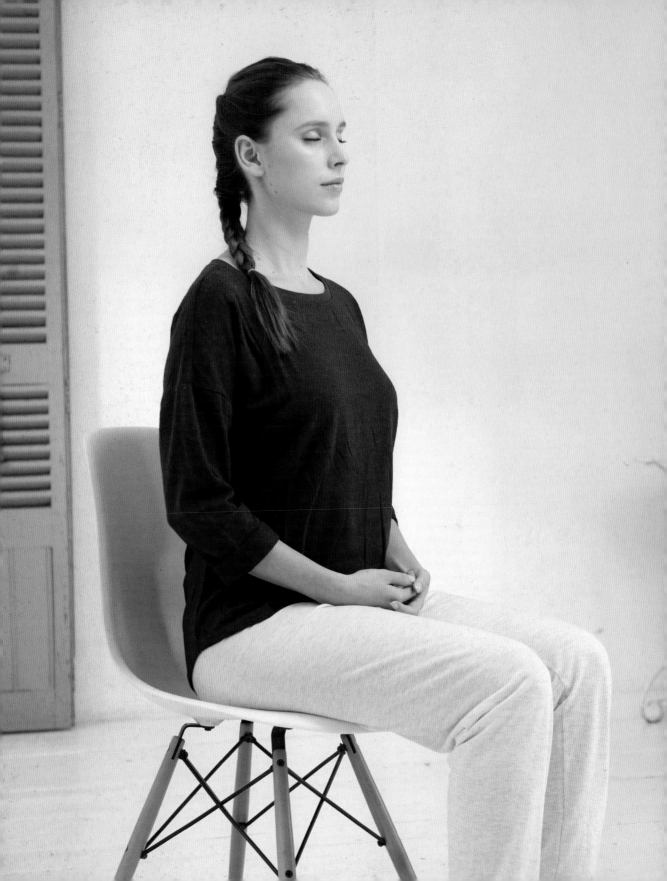

# Introduction

Welcome to Body in Mind Training – a unique approach to mindfulness that uses the moving body as the primary learning tool. My intention in this book is to share with you the techniques I have discovered in the course of my own personal and professional journey toward a happier, healthier, more integrated self. My approach, which combines meditation with martial arts and neuroscience, is designed to be accessible to anyone, including those who struggle with traditional sitting meditation or who can't seem to find the time in their busy schedules to practise.

## How are you, right now?

Take a minute to congratulate yourself on finding some time in your busy schedule to open this book. Now pause for a second, in this very moment, and simply breathe. What does your body really feel like? Where is your mind right now? Is your attention here in the present moment, or has it already wandered off somewhere, into the past or the future?

If you're anything like me, your mind is constantly active – judging, comparing, planning, analysing, ruminating and remembering. We are so busy thinking, thinking, thinking all day long. We field and respond to endless emails, phone calls, obligations, responsibilities, fears, worries, to-do lists and chores. Even in our sleep, most of us don't really switch off.

All this is hardly surprising given the fast-paced technological world we now live in. Our overworked minds are constantly bombarded with distractions and stimuli at every turn. We don't know where to focus our attention first, as we rush from place to place and task to task. We keep thinking harder, in a desperate attempt to try to manage our brain's overloaded inbox. There are simply never enough hours in the day to get everything done. Slow down? No way! In fact, for most of us, the very thought of slowing down is terrifying.

Yet the way we live comes at a huge cost, both to our bodies and our minds. We become disconnected and out of balance, and we lose sight of where we are heading. At worst, this results in mental and physical illness. At best, our life just flashes by in the blink of an eye, as we operate on a mindless autopilot, week in–week out. Before we know it, ten years have passed us by.

So what would it be like to have more time and space in your life for the things that really matter?

How can you still your busy mind so you can see and think more clearly? Imagine living a life of ease and joy, no matter what challenges you encounter.

In your dreams, right? But what if I told you that this spaciousness and freedom really is possible for all of us? What if I told you it lies in your ability to connect more fully to the present moment; that it exists in a wonderful way of being that we call 'mindfulness'?

I will guide you step by step through my Body in Mind Training (BMT) programme, a unique approach to secular mindfulness practice that uses the moving body as the main meditation tool. This pioneering approach has arisen from my unique perspective working not only as a published neuroscientist and practising clinical psychologist, but also as a mindfulness trainer; it is a culmination of decades of research, clinical study and practice, and mindfulness teaching, which has taken me across the globe.

Operating at the forefront of the disciplines of neuroscience, psychology and martial arts – not just as an academic and clinician but also as a lecturer, trainer and practitioner – has given me a huge advantage in the continually evolving field of secular mindfulness, and one for which I feel immensely privileged and grateful.

I hope that as I share some of my expertise and knowledge in this book, you too will be inspired to engage with your body and mind in a new and different way, one that will bring about the lasting changes you are seeking in your life. I will attempt to show you how, with a little focus, determination and practice, you too can experience the amazing benefits of mindfulness. All it takes on your part is the courage and curiosity to do something different – a willingness to have a go.

# Body in Mind Training

This body-based brain-training technique uses mindful movement (moving meditation, in other words) to keep us anchored in the present moment. Central to BMT is the belief that the body and the mind are intimately connected.

T raditionally, in the West, body and mind have been viewed as separate entities. This perspective has been challenged in recent years, including by the emerging field of embodied cognitive neuroscience.[1] Research from mindfulness training studies also supports the notion that the former 'poor cousin' – the body – may in fact be more of a key player in our conscious experience than we ever previously imagined.[2] Taking this one step further, we are now beginning to understand how the movement of the body affects the movement of the mind[3] (a fascinating concept we will explore in more detail later). This new scientific insight has far-reaching implications both for the development of medical science and for our general approach to wellbeing, not least the advancement of mindfulness theory and practice.

BMT involves paying full attention, moment by moment, to the sensations of the moving body, as a precursor to developing the ability to detect far subtler movements of the mind. The insights we gain as we observe our moving body enables us to see more clearly the origins of all our actions and reactions. With greater awareness, we can choose to act in ways that tap into our innate wisdom, rather than running our lives on autopilot.

The BMT message is a simple one: getting out of your head and into your body is the key to a happier, healthier life. The problem for all of us today is that we are trying to solve most of life's problems in our heads, using our thinking minds. But what if I were to tell you that the solution lies not so much in your head, but more in your body? Your body is talking to you all the time. But in order to hear it, you have to slow down and listen to its voice – and this is the starting point for BMT mindfulness practice. I hope that my easy-to-follow and practical guide to mindful movement will give you all the tools you need to become more connected, Body in MInd.

Over the years, when discussing the BMT approach with friends, colleagues and clients, I've noticed the first thing they say is, 'but isn't it body *and* mind?' However, it is clear to me that it has to be body *in* mind, because body and mind are not separate, they operate as one.

The BMT message is a simple one: getting out of your head and into your body is the key to a happier, healthier life!

## The BMT story

For years, alongside my neuroscience studies, I trained in the martial art of Shaolin kung fu. When I reached the black belt level, I became really aware of just what I could achieve when training at the mind–body interface. Training at this level is a way to engage with and challenge all those mental and emotional blocks that hold us back in life. Yet aspects of the physical training in martial arts can be punishing – designed to break down the ego and bring the body right to the edge. It wasn't until a few years later, when I moved into internal martial arts, training in tai chi ch'uan, that I learned it is also possible to engage with the body and mind in a kinder, more compassionate way, and with far less chance of injury.

A few years later, as a trainee clinical psychologist at University College London, I found that tai chi helped me to stay centred and calm, even in those moments of panic when I was faced with a very distressed client. I began to notice that through my tai chi practice I was developing a body awareness that was actually helping me to connect with my clients at a far deeper level. The notion that becoming more bodily aware (or 'embodied') profoundly benefits the client–therapist relationship began to fascinate me.[4]

It was during my early academic career, while studying experimental psychology (specifically, social cognition), that I began to ask myself the fundamental questions that would go on to shape the early design of the BMT programme: 'Is it possible to bring brain processes that usually lie outside awareness into awareness using our attention?' And: 'Would this make a difference to those who struggle with social cognition and have difficulties in life as a result?' Published in 2008, my research showed that training in social cognition *was* possible and gave individuals with severe mental illness and difficulties with social situations the confidence to engage more in social activities, vastly improving their quality of life.[5]

Around the same time, when I was undertaking post-doctorate research into social cognition at Macquarie University, Sydney, I met an Australian woman who was to change the course of my life. Interacting with her, you would never guess she had received a childhood diagnosis of schizophrenia and suffered chronic auditory hallucinations. I was curious as to how she was managing to live such a full life, including working and living independently. She told me that she had discovered the work of Jon Kabat-Zinn, the founder of secular mindfulness, and since then had practised mindfulness every day. She described how mindfulness training helped her to distinguish the predominately negative voices related to her illness from the supportive voices of her Maori spiritual tradition. Her story made me realize that mindfulness might be able to help the people with similar difficulties I was encountering in my clinical psychology practice.

I was keen to find out if it was possible to integrate martial arts training principles that use the moving body with psychological theory to help people who might normally struggle with traditional talking therapies, or to sit still. For example, would such integration help people with a diagnosis of schizophrenia or other conditions in which the mind is extremely chaotic? I mused that a more body-

I began to explore new ways of utilizing the moving body to facilitate, accelerate and deepen the mindfulness training experience.

orientated moving approach might be a better route to symptom management and inner healing. I began to experiment, designing the first BMT prototype exercises and framework.

Around this time research was proving that mindfulness training, in particular the MBSR (Mindfulness Based Stress Reduction) and MBCT (Mindfulness Based Cognitive Therapy) programmes devised by Jon Kabat-Zinn and colleagues at Massachusetts University, and by Mark Williams and colleagues at Oxford University, were really helping people with chronic pain and recurring mental health conditions such as clinical anxiety and depression.[6] I discovered that the Body Scan – where the practitioner is repeatedly asked to bring attention to different parts of the body while lying down, completely still – was a critical part of these programmes. At the same time I was also aware from my own academic work that brain-imaging studies were showing structural changes in the regions of the brain related to the body and its movement, and that mindful movement practice is highly correlated with increased mindfulness and self compassion.[7]

This prompted further questions: 'What more can we learn from the moving body?' 'How might the moving body inform and enhance the development of mindfulness practice in the West?' And: 'How might this benefit people who would otherwise struggle with the formal seated practices and programmes through lack of time or other constraints?'

Inspired, I began to explore new ways of utilizing the moving body to facilitate, accelerate and deepen the mindfulness training experience, using what I had learned from my neuroscience and martial arts backgrounds to create a new and easier way to meditate. BMT was born!

## What happened next

The results of the first BMT groups I ran for patients and staff in psychiatric settings back in 2006 were encouraging. It was amazing to observe how even those with very challenging and distressed mental states could attain a sense of calm and relaxation through mindful movement exercises alone.[8]

Over time, I gradually developed the BMT workshops for a much broader client base, including mental healthcare workers, doctors and nurses, as well as people in education, sports, corporate settings, prisons and the arts. With each workshop, I experimented with different practices, listened to responses, observed reactions and reflected on the insights I gained. All the exercises you are about to learn have been refined through years of these group training sessions; all have been used by a wide variety of participants from around the world.[9]

With such diverse groups to work with, I soon realized that there was a lot of confusion about mindfulness as a concept, from the terminology to the training methods. That's why I set out to create an easy and pragmatic guide to mindfulness practice – something that would be more accessible for the average person.

## Who is this book for?

If you struggle with the idea of sitting still for sustained periods to meditate, BMT can provide you with a manageable alternative. This approach is for anyone who would like to experience the benefits of mindfulness practice in their lives – even for those of us who are *really* busy. Because the moving body is with you all the time, you can practise the exercises almost anywhere and at any time throughout your demanding day.

## Why BMT is different

People often ask me to describe the difference between my BMT programme and the traditional MBSR and MBCT training programmes.

Essentially, my BMT framework is based on the same classic meditation theory as MBSR, but there are some major differences in the delivery and teaching method. The five components of the BMT programme – Pause, Intention, Attention, Understanding me, and Compassion – arose from unpacking Jon Kabat-Zinn's standard definition, which states that mindfulness is 'the awareness that arises from paying attention, on purpose, moment by moment and non-judgmentally'.[10]

I offer people multiple entry points to mindfulness in the hope that they will find the path that is right for them.

The more traditional programmes such as MBSR use static postures as the main tool to train attention and observe the impermanence of bodily and mental sensations – and so the impermanence of life itself. There is a strong emphasis on staying with the experience and continuing practice, with little overt theory. This is a Zen-style training method many Westerners find hard to engage with.

The five components of the BMT programme

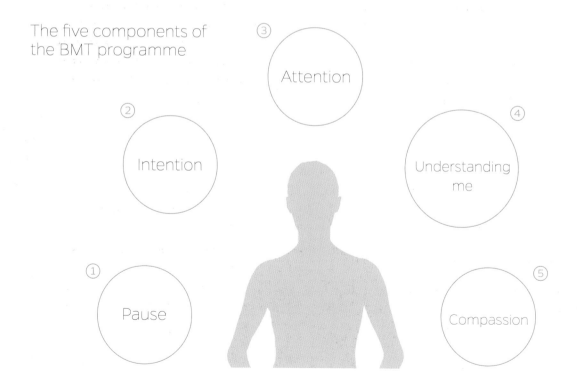

③ Attention

② Intention

④ Understanding me

① Pause

⑤ Compassion

BMT balances practical learning with conceptual learning. Primarily, we use the moving body to train us in the detection of movement of mind, and back up each exercise with insights from cutting-edge neuroscience. For some people this extra understanding of why we are doing something can really help to increase motivation.

I do not profess the BMT programme to be the only route to mindfulness practice. Nor am I suggesting that this route is for everyone. And I am certainly not challenging in any way the efficacy and brilliance of the mainstream secular MBSR and MBCT programmes – these programmes have a huge role to play.

Rather, the BMT system provides an alternative way to connect to mindfulness primarily through the moving body. I offer people multiple entry points to the practice – through marital arts, mindfulness theory and neuroscience – in the hope that they will find the path that is right for them.

This book represents my current understanding of mindfulness as it relates to my own life and work. While I draw on ancient traditions, my secular variant of mindfulness is constantly evolving. And, like everyone else, I still have much to learn about how body, brain and mind interconnect.

## BMT today

BMT has been the subject of a number of successful pilot studies[11], at King's College London[12], for example, and some larger international research studies are underway. BMT has been delivered to elite athletes at the University of the West Indies, as well as being implemented in schools, business and healthcare settings in the UK, Brazil, Poland and Barbados. Participants report that the combination of a neuroscientific understanding, alongside really practical things that they can do *right now* with their bodies and body awareness, make BMT a highly pragmatic approach to mindfulness training.

While I recognize the value of empirical research, I am interested most of all in the personal stories of transformation that I hear about every day as part of my work. These reports come from people who have completed BMT training.

The practice

## Working with the moving body

Many people question whether meditating on the moving body can really deliver the same benefits as sitting quietly on a cushion; 'Surely the whole point is that you have to be still,' they say. However, in tai chi philosophy and practice the notion of exploring the mind through the body is the same as in any still meditation practice. For me, there are many extra benefits that arise from working with the moving body, including:

○ Your moving body is with you all the time, so you can meditate anywhere.

○ Learning through the body deepens and facilitates your experience.

○ Detecting movement in the motor domain helps you to recognize mental movement patterns more easily.

○ Movement keeps you physically healthy.

# How to use this book

The BMT programme has been designed to help people practise mindfulness anywhere, at any time. It combines two strands of learning: one that focuses on the body, through practical exercises, and one that engages the brain.

E ven if you work only with one strand of the practice, you will derive benefit, but for the best results from BMT, I urge you to work with both of these approaches:

① **Practical learning through the body** A series of carefully designed movement exercises will enable you to learn the principles of mindfulness through the body. This is known as embodied learning.

② **Conceptual learning via the brain** Information and observations drawn from mindfulness theory, martial arts theory and neuroscience will support your practical experience.

## How the book is organized

The book is divided into six chapters, starting with an explanation of mindful movement and why it can greatly enhance your mindfulness practice. In developing BMT, I have taken the standard definition of mindfulness and organized it into five main training principles – Pause, Intention, Attention, Understanding me, and Compassion. These principles form the structure of the programme and I've dedicated a chapter to each one.

In **Chapter 1 (A new way to meditate)** I explain what mindfulness is and how the BMT method sits alongside other, more traditional mindfulness techniques, such as those found in Zen Buddhism and tai chi.

In **Chapter 2 (Pause)** I explore the concept of pausing – the starting point for all mindfulness practice. I show you how slowing down your internal pace can help you to enter the present moment and how learning to put the brakes on your body and therefore on your brain can help you live with more skill and ease.

In **Chapter 3 (Intention)** I'll show you how setting your intention in your brain before you act can dramatically increase your ability to stay on track and achieve what you want in life.

In **Chapter 4 (Attention)** you'll learn to detect the mind-wandering habits that hold you back in life, and discover how to widen and narrow your lens of attention in order to create more space in your mind, and to increase your capacity for sustained concentration.

In **Chapter 5 (Understanding me)** I'll help you to delve deeper to gain greater insight into how your mind really works. I'll show you how to manage your unruly habits of mind (we call them 'mental monkeys') and create new neural pathways that help you to realize your full potential.

In **Chapter 6 (Compassion)**, the last chapter, I'll show you how body awareness can increase your capacity for compassion. You'll learn how facing and accepting difficult experiences can profoundly transform your relationship with life. I'll explain how to engage with the centres of empathy and compassion in your brain in order to live with more joy and peace.

In every chapter you'll find insights from mindfulness, neuroscience and martial arts. I've provided these to deepen your understanding of mindfulness and enhance your training experience. Chapter by chapter, a series of brain-training exercises encourages you to practise on a regular basis, because the more you practise, the easier BMT gets. Try to embrace the exercises with as little expectation as possible.

> In any tai chi practice session, I explore all five aspects of BMT. I slow down, move with intention, pay attention, learn about myself and find out how powerful ease and gentleness can be.

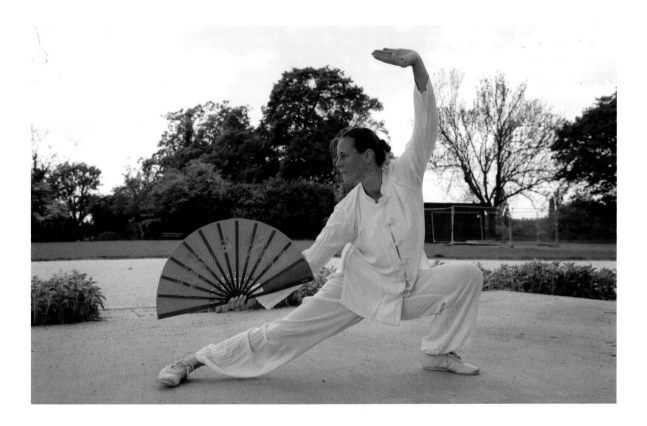

**Let's practise** exercises are designed to give you a direct body-based experience of a key training concept. You can practise many of them formally as part of a daily training programme or informally as you mix and match to suit your needs. Practise them on a regular basis for the best results.

At the end of some of these exercises are **Be curious** boxes, which include variations on the main exercise to help you explore the sensations and experiences of that exercise more fully or in different ways.

**Have a go** exercises are short and quick and intended for you to try right here, right now – just put the book down and have a go.

**Reflect on this** boxes are invitations to think about how you might apply the mindfulness principles to your wider life to help you see and act differently. Be playful and experiment with the ideas I've given as much as possible.

As you explore the book, there are also two important concepts that you need to bear in mind:

(1) **The eyes of a child**, which in martial arts is how we invite you to see the world. Try to drop your adult expectations and ask yourself, 'How would a child engage with this experience? What would it be like to observe this for the first time?' Cultivate internally and intentionally this stance of wide-eyed curiosity and openness and maintain it throughout your training (it's very easy to allow it to slip away – hold on to it). As you practise you'll discover that even though you sometimes think you already 'know' something, there is still much for you to learn.

(2) **Keeping a balance** between the conceptual and practical learning. While it is important that the latest neuroscience research informs your understanding of what is going on in your brain, getting too wedded to the notion that it is all about the science is likely to inhibit your progress. This book is about developing a balance between science, consciousness and the moving body. The multiple entry points are designed to help you find your own way to a healthy and satisfying practice.

## Why you need to practise

Culturally, we tend to look for quick results – to find the answer in the pages of a book or on the Internet. This search for a quick fix is also spreading into mindfulness practice, with more and more ideas floating around about how to learn quickly to live in the moment.

But just as reading innumerable magazines on how to lose weight won't actually reduce your waistline, so reading book after book on mindfulness won't rewire your brain's neural pathways. You need to engage in some practice to actually succeed.

There is ongoing debate about the relative benefits of formal practice (dedicated times when you engage with mindfulness practice no matter what) and informal practice (finding moments in your life that you can make mindful). I believe that both have a place in our lives, but if you are at the start of your mindfulness journey, the martial arts principle of 'kung fu is everything you do' applies – you will

> It's really crucial in mindfulness training to let your inner child come to the fore and cultivate an attitude of curiosity and openness.

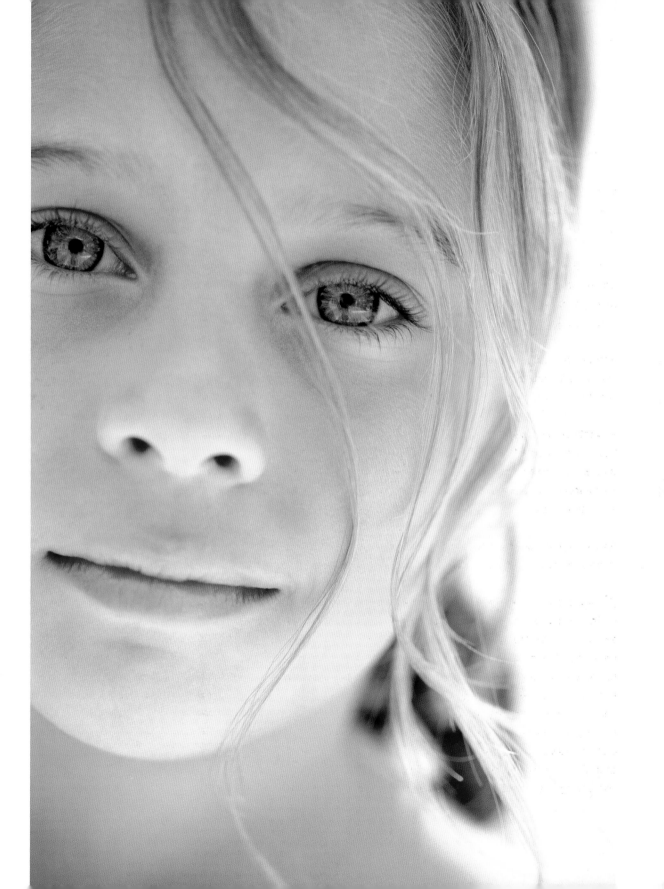

## A starting point

Defining the word 'mindfulness' is problematic, let alone getting into terms such as 'consciousness' and 'mind'. Even today, after millennia of exploration in the spiritual workings of the mind, Buddhist scholars, translators, cognitive scientists and philosophers continue to argue over the definition of mindfulness. I am not a contemplative scholar, nor even a student or philosopher in the field of consciousness, although, of course, I am fascinated by mindfulness and its many strands. In this book, I will attempt to provide you with some broad definitions to get you started. Please note that there are many excellent sources of teachings and knowledge, and this book represents my own understanding of ancient texts and modern psychological concepts and how these relate to each other. If you find a reference in this book to another work that might inspire you, I urge you to seek it out and discover its teachings so that you can explore all the theories and concepts in whatever ways interest you most.

certainly get some benefit from engaging mindfully in your daily activities and I encourage you to start in whatever ways you can.

### How to practise

Most importantly, have fun! Try to engage with BMT in a playful, lighthearted way. The mind is such a crazy place for us all and humour makes remaining sane seem so much easier. See if you can really 'smile from the heart' as you complete each practice. If you are not able to practise for whatever reason, or you notice a dip in your motivation, try reading around the subject to re-inspire you. Try watching a kung fu movie or some tai chi videos to keep moving forward in some way. Although there is no substitute for regular, physical practice, it's okay to be kind to yourself sometimes – simply engage in whatever is possible for you, in that moment. There is no right or wrong way, so just find the path that works for you.

I hope that the accessibility of my BMT method – the exercises combined with the mindfulness theory and accompanying brain science – will inspire and motivate you to keep practising. However, the most important learning tool comes in the 'doing' – actually getting into the postures, and revisiting the exercises over and over again.

Here are some answers to some of the most frequently asked questions …

**Do I need a cushion?** No! Seated practices offer great value, but they can also be daunting in terms both of mental challenge and physical discomfort. I have designed this mindful movement training guide so that you can practise meditation anytime, anywhere – without a cushion!

**What if I feel pain?** Some people may experience discomfort or pain while doing these exercises. This is not a reason to stop, but could be a reason to modify them. If the pain is related to a past or current injury, you may need to adapt the exercise slightly to your ability. Reconnecting with your body can make low-level aches and pains more apparent. Part of the mindful learning process is getting in touch with sensations that you have (consciously or unconsciously) avoided, denied or suppressed, opening up your awareness to what is really there and choosing to engage with it fully. Mindful movement should rarely result in injury, as you are starting slowly and paying full attention. Pay attention to any tightness or pain, find your own limits and be gentle with yourself. Straining or striving indicates this is no longer mindful movement. Go slowly and bring a kind, curious attention to any sensations you experience. From awareness comes skilful action.

If you do suffer any pain during your practice, consider whether there is an opportunity for you to learn something about your body before you dull it with painkillers. Be extremely curious about what happens in your mind as you experience pain, including thoughts such as 'I can't do it', 'This will harm me' or 'I should stop.' These thoughts are often habitual and are likely to be directly impacting your physical experience. Try your best not to get too caught up in them and stay with the physical sensations – exploring the edges of the pain and the regions nearby. Meditate on the affected body part and find out as much as possible, determining from the inside where your pain stops and starts, the types of sensation (stabbing or throbbing, for example) and the edges of your pain. Note any mental reactions, such as loss, grief or a desire for things to be different.

**What if I don't feel anything?** At first, many people find it hard to locate sensations in their body. If this is the case for you, don't give up. It's possible that your mind is so busy thinking, analysing and planning that your body can't get a word in edgeways. Over time, you'll find it easier to calm your chattering mind long enough to develop enhanced sensitivity to your body's sensations. In the meantime, choose a practice that allows you to turn your mind's eye to a body part

## Note of caution

## Seeking help

Body in Mind Training (BMT) can bring about massive and lasting changes in both mental and physical wellbeing, helping you to unlock your own healing potential and make profound changes in your life. You may be able to do far more for yourself than you think. However, this book is not meant to be a substitute for professional medical or psychological help. Although the BMT approach and exercises will certainly augment and complement other treatments, it is wise to know when professional help is necessary.

that evokes a lot of sensations – your hands or face, for example – or simply conduct the movement more slowly and deliberately to evoke more sensation.

### Let's go!

BMT gives you the choice and flexibility to learn mindfulness via both the thinking (conceptual) route and the practical (experiential) route. You can choose to explore mindful movement freely as you go about your day, or you can choose to use it in a formal practice for which you deliberately put aside time to engage with your moving body. I hope that this multipronged, free-flowing framework enables you to explore mindfulness whatever your commitments and available time, and find a way to make it work for you.

So, it just now remains for me to wish you well as you embark on your transformational mindfulness journey. This journey promises to be at once illuminating, interesting and surprising, and perhaps even a little challenging at times. May curiosity, courage and compassion be always at your side.

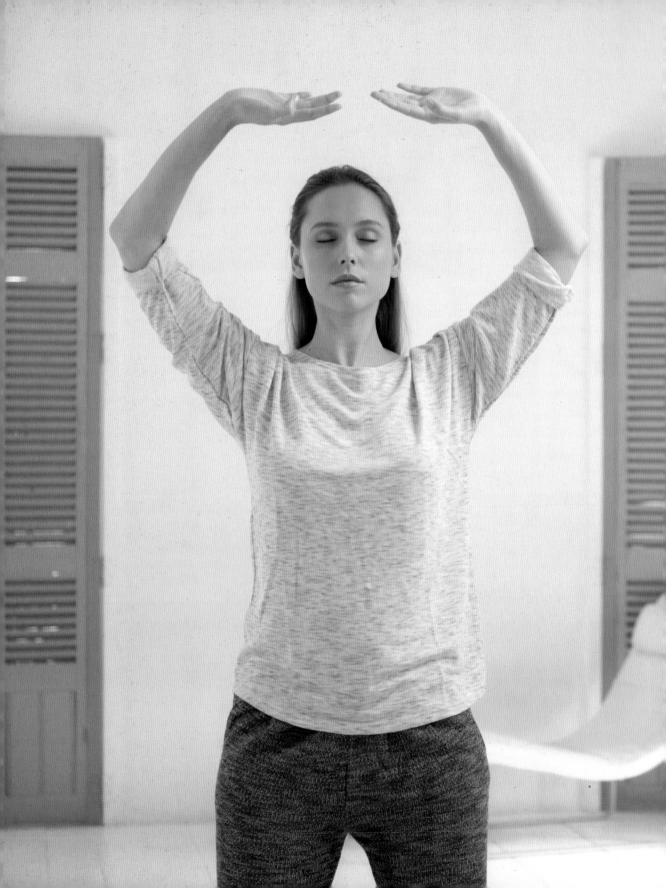

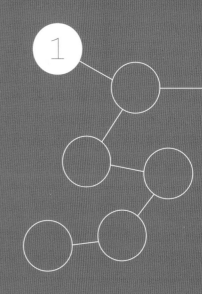

1

# A new way to meditate

Mindfulness has been part of contemplative traditions such as Buddhism for thousands of years, but it is only in the last four decades that it has entered our mainstream Western life, thanks to the work of Jon Kabat-Zinn and others. These days the word is part of everyday language – you can hardly open a paper or a magazine without reading about mindfulness. Yet it is still considered by many only as a *mental* training. In fact, the practice of mindfulness starts with attending to the body,[1] becoming intimate with our bodily sensations and then using these to learn more about how the mind works. Working with the moving body helps to facilitate and deepen our learning experience.[2]

# Your body and your mind

The benefits of mindfulness are well established, with corporate giants now offering meditation training in the workplace.[3] But what if you can't find the time for formal daily practice? And what if your mind is so busy that even sitting still for just five minutes seems impossible?

F our decades of research into the standard eight-week MBSR (Mindfulness Based Stress Reduction)[4] programme, and more recently into MBCT (Mindfulness Based Cognitive Therapy)[5] have demonstrated that mindfulness provides enormous physical and mental health benefits. These exist not only for those for whom the programmes were originally intended (people with chronic physical ailments whose treatment had reached the limits of the medical model in the case of MBSR, and those with recurrent mental health challenges such as major depression in the case of MBCT), but for all people in all walks of life.

However, such mindfulness courses, although extremely effective, ask participants to make significant lifestyle changes requiring great motivation and engagement. What options are there for those of us who are suffering less, but might still like to enjoy the benefits of mindfulness?

## What is mindful movement?

A form of moving meditation, mindful movement engages full awareness of intention, attention and all our physical and mental sensations as they unfold over time. It is conducted with a stance of compassionate acceptance toward each and every sensation – whether a thought, feeling, memory, emotion or bodily sensation.

Throughout this book the primary focus is on the way your brain detects movement at multiple levels – movement of your limbs, of your emotions, of your attention and of your mind. If you can become an expert at detecting movement throughout your body, you can access the stillness that lies within you.

Physical movement unfolds over time – it has a beginning, a middle and an end. Neuroscience research tells us that temporal sequences occur in the mind, too. These help to order our thoughts and execute our plans in a logical order. When we are stressed, not being able to 'think straight' is often the first thing that we notice, a reflection of how this ordering process is lost.

Bodily movement gives us more concrete sensations to attend to while we're training, which is particularly helpful when you're new to the practice. If you can practise paying attention to your moving body, learning how to detect subtle differences in

Sitting meditation is the traditional way of accessing inner stillness, yet some people may find being still for even short periods of time too challenging.

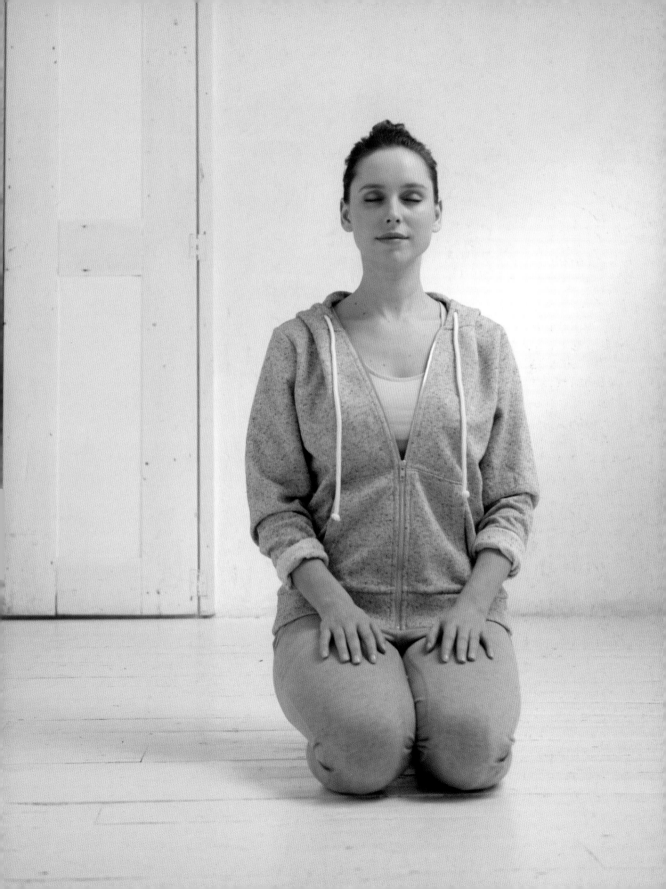

pace and timing, you'll gradually learn to tap into the more subtle sensations occurring in your mind.

Your thoughts, feelings and emotions are part of a long chain of mental and physical sensations, all of them transient – arising and fading away, if you let them be. My belief is that understanding the connections between body and mind in this way improves the interrelationship between thoughts, feelings and actions in the wider world. Your body, and how you use it, control it and relate to it, offers tremendous insight into the workings of your mind.

The end result is to improve dramatically your emotional capabilities and mental resilience in the face of challenge, and to help you manage difficult or emotional states, including chronic mental pain.

## Movement and cognition

We know that movement and cognition (understanding) are intimately linked, and numerous studies have shown the positive effects that physical exercise can have on cognition.[7] We also know that practising sequences of movement changes the structure of our highly 'plastic' brains.[8]

Latest advances in neuroscience also highlight the importance of the body's motor system in our understanding of learning and brain development.[9] Neuroscientist and movement expert Daniel Wolpert[10] believes that the reason the human brain developed as it did was primarily to resolve problems we encountered as we began to move about our environment. So, the processes that co-ordinate, execute and regulate movement are the building blocks for the mental processes that co-ordinate, execute and regulate so-called higher order functions, such as thinking and emotional experience.

## Movement and mood

Clinical studies tell us that age-related movement disorders, for example Parkinson's Disease, and depression often occur together, leading neuroscientists to conclude that when we don't move, we feel low. We also know that the most effective treatment for mild to moderate depression (as effective as anti-depressants) is to go for a walk or to do some exercise, and there may be a particular case to be made for meditative movement such as tai chi.[11]

Movement is also linked to mood and motivation in as much as we move toward things we like and away from things we don't. This hard-wiring forms the basis of all our behaviour, whether it's a physical movement toward or away from, or a mental one – that is, whether we engage with (approach) or avoid thoughts, feelings, emotions or bodily sensations. Becoming familiar with these push/pull movements through the BMT exercises helps our understanding of our most basic motivations and emotions.

Brain science

## Parallel development

When infants begin to explore the world through movement, many cognitive and social-processing abilities begin to emerge.[6] Their memory improves and they become better able to deal with spatial problems and perceive what's going on around them. At the other end of life, research tells us that changes in the gait of older adults are predictive of the onset of neurodegenerative diseases, such as Parkinson's Disease. It appears that how we are in our body is representative of our internal experience.

# The moving practices

The biggest difference between BMT and classes teaching traditional moving practices, such as martial arts, is that right from the start BMT brings all movements into full awareness, attending to the movements of your mind as well as your body.

T he underlying principles of mindful movement are the same as those in seated mindfulness. Both train the mind *to pay attention, on purpose and without judgment, to what is occurring in each moment.* In BMT, however, we focus on the *moving* body.

While it is true that most traditional moving practices, such tai chi and chi kung, can help to balance body and mind, progress can be excruciatingly slow. Classes typically rely on the repetition of sequences of moves, manual correction of posture from the teacher, and little in the way of overt instruction of the mental experience. The learning emerges through the body. Many people leave tai chi classes before they get to the learning part because the slow nature of the practice does not sit well with the Western mindset.

In BMT classes we try to conduct every single movement, adjustment and exploration with full mindful awareness – observing the intention, the execution and the unfolding sensory consequences of each movement, as well as remaining aware of other mental sensations (thoughts, feelings, memories, images) as they unfold.

Engaging in simple mindful movement practices on a regular basis can dramatically alter your experience of the world. Martial arts and other Eastern body-based traditions, such as yoga and tai chi, have at their heart the premise that movement, posture and bodily awareness shape consciousness.

The student's response to the challenges of working with the body in new and demanding ways reveals intimate links between body and mind. Some exercises are designed to be particularly provocative, enabling the teacher to observe quickly the psychological state of the student. This body–mind interface is interrogated further as you reach advanced levels.

In both BMT and martial arts practice, we create sensations in order to work with them – for example, you might deliberately make a movement in order to help you connect to an experience. This is a very different approach to traditional mindfulness practices, such as the MBSR programme, which are more informed by the Zen approach. Zen practices tend to avoid creating sensations, guiding students instead to 'just watch' what arises naturally. It is important to remember that there is no right or wrong way to connect to mindfulness practice – from Zen to tai chi to BMT, these are all just different training techniques. The important thing is that you know what you are doing and why you are doing it.

# BMT and embodied learning

In BMT, and in the exercises in this book, I use an approach known as 'embodied learning', which literally means 'learning through the body'. This recognizes that a different and more efficient type of learning experience is possible when we engage our whole mind–body system.

In embodied learning, concepts such as *'opening to experience'* or *'dropping thoughts'* are not abstract, but are experienced directly through the configuration of the moving body – we feel and see them. This approach deepens our learning experience, as we are engaging much more than just our 'thinking' brain. Have you ever referred to someone *grasping* what you were saying? Or said that you are *leaning* toward doing something? These are both linguistic examples of embodied learning: body-action verbs describing a cognitive (thinking) process.

## Embodiment and the consciousness debate

The term 'embodiment'[12] is currently experiencing something of a resurgence in philosophical, cognitive and neuroscience fields, particularly in debates about the nature of consciousness. Despite many decades of research, we have made little progress in our attempts to understand this by focusing on the brain alone. The scientific community is now opening to the idea that embodied cognition has something to offer the biggest philosophical question – what is consciousness? The definition of 'embodiment' is controversial, but I draw on the work of Rosch,

Thompson and Varela[13] for inspiration, who consider embodied cognition to apply to the way the body and the brain both interact with a person's environment and work together to create conscious experience.

Is the mind in the brain? Contemplative scholar B Alan Wallace has written a number of excellent articles and books that address this fascinating and tricky philosophical question, examining the Buddhist view of the mind, and modern conceptualizations of mind and brain[14].

Brain science

## Benefits of embodied learning

Learning through your moving body enables you to draw on a more widely distributed network of brain regions, engaging more of your brain in your learning. It also allows you to see in a concrete way mental patterns such as 'holding' or 'tightening', as well as what it's like to 'open' or 'let go' – the types of movements we aspire to in the mind. Seeing patterns in the body helps you to identifiy them when you meet them in the abstract realm of the mind, enabling you to stop them in their tracks and modify thoughts and behaviour to take more positive action.

On-going dialogue between contemplative practitioners and cognitive scientists, such as that promoted by the Mind and Life Institute[15], is helping us to find out more about the connection between brain and mind. For example, early psychologists found introspective approaches yielded unreliable data and discontinued this line of enquiry. However, attentional training methods developed by Eastern contemplatives provide a key to access this chaotic inner experience in a structured way.

My tai chi training leans me toward views held by authors such as Varela, who suggests that mind extends beyond brain into the body and the wider environment. Tai chi practice, particularly when done in the natural environment, allows us to really feel the connection between our physical movements, our mental movements and the ever-changing movements observed in nature and all around us. In this way, the meditative movements of tai chi can help us to understand the interconnectedness of all things.

Open-air meditative exercise, like this session in Hangzhou, China, can really help us to explore the interconnection of our mind, body and environment.

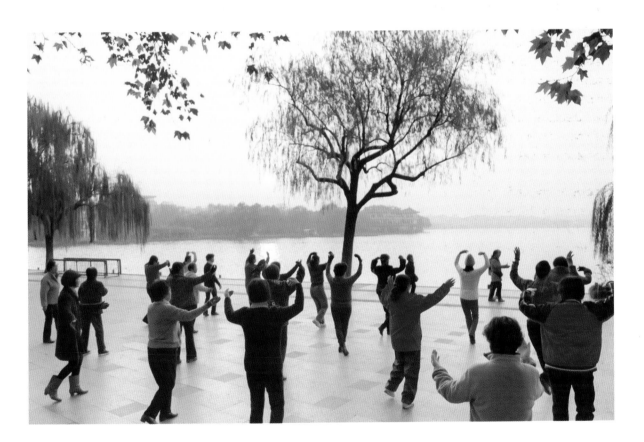

# BMT and neuroscience

Embedded in the design and delivery of the BMT programme is knowledge about how the brain works. My work as a researcher and lecturer and my neuroscience knowledge inform the choice of exercises and how I teach them.

M y aim is to make the insights of the practice more obvious to participants, giving them an easily observable and direct experience of their brains, increasing the learning potential as a result.

Drawing on information about numerous other brains that have been involved in scientific studies helps us to see that we are not alone in our experiences, and that each of our mental and physical experiences is not something that should make us feel fearful or overwhelmed – they are simply a consequence of what the brain does.

Recent research indicates that our brains are much more malleable than was first thought[16]. Several studies show that we can change both the structure and function of key brain regions that are related to attention and emotion regulation through mindfulness training[17]. Even as fully grown adults it's possible to rewire connections in the brain. This neuroplasticity has been repeatedly demonstrated in relation to motor learning[18] and now is beginning to

be shown as resulting from the internal, attentional training of mindfulness[19].

Neuroscience is used in a few ways in the BMT approach. First, BMT takes what is known about how the brain is organized to guide the development of exercises, selecting those that tap directly into the brain structures that will provide the most consistent and concrete learning experiences. For example, Chapter 4 includes exercises that work with the face and hands, as the regions of the brain dedicated to these areas are larger than those focused on other body parts (see page 79).

Secondly, BMT selects exercises that engage with brain processes in a way that can be clearly observed through the body (for example, we inhibit physical movements in order to regulate emotions – see pages 45–7). Finally, sharing this information with the interested learner is, in my experience, a key motivator that promotes curiosity and engagement. The majority of my students have commented that it has really helped them to understand more about the neuroscience behind the exercises.

Having said all that, it's worth emphasizing that it's not all about the science! This book is an attempt to redress our tendency to live in our minds, helping you to discover the benefits of reconnecting to your body.

Even as fully grown adults it's possible to rewire connections in the brain.

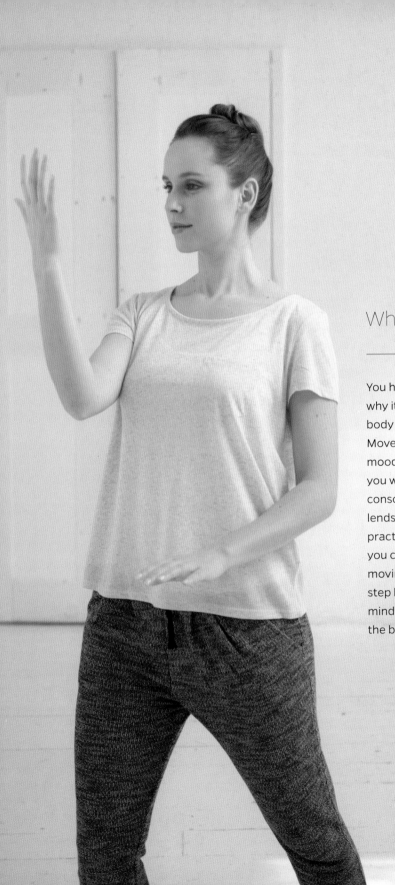

## Where you are now

You have discovered some of the reasons why it might be a good idea to use the moving body as your main mindfulness training tool. Movement is intimately connected with your mood and your thinking, and can provide you with an alternative route to explore your conscious experiences. The moving body also lends a richness and depth to your mindfulness practice. And, best of all, this approach means you can practise mindfulness any time you are moving! The following chapters will take you step by step through a process of developing mindfulness skills via exercises that work with the body.

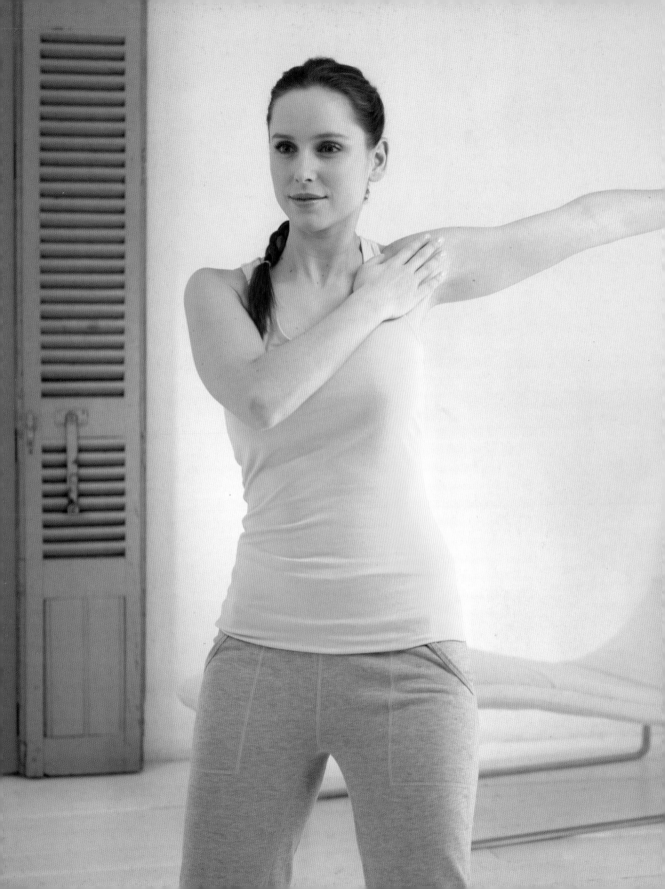

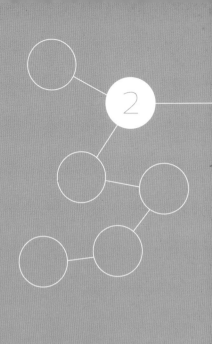

# Pause

Central to mindfulness training is learning to keep our attention on what is happening right now, in the present moment; not getting stuck in the past or rushing into the future. When we are ruminating, caught up in worry and anxious thinking, we are not really 'here' and we miss so much of what is happening in and around us. But where is this present moment? How do we get there? And how do we stay there? In this chapter you'll learn two simple but effective methods for accessing the present moment: the first is pausing; the second, 'dropping into the body'. Even the most recent research in the field of neuroscience now suggests that mindfulness starts with the body.[1]

# The challenge of slowing down

When I suggest to people (and myself!) to slow down, the response is often, 'How can I possibly slow down? There is so much to do and so little time! To stop would be madness!' However, we often have to learn the hard way that pushing on can damage both body and mind.

E verything seems to be working against us when we try to slow down. Thanks in particular to modern technology, the pace of life today can seem relentless. We can all feel captive to our cell phones, tablets, laptops; and disconnecting is not easy – even just thinking about it can make some people feel anxious! This has given rise to the idea of separation anxiety from our gadgets.[2] The speed and ubiquity of this information flow perpetuates future-oriented states of mind, disconnects us from our bodies and often leads to increased anxiety.

### Doing less is doing more!

Although it feels counterintuitive, times of 'too much to do' are exactly when you need to pause – and just breathe. Paradoxically, slowing down and pausing actually give us more in our lives, not less, because

## Connect with nature

Find some pictures of natural scenes to put on your computer and observe what happens in your body when you look at them. If you have a chance, cut through a park or communal garden as you travel to or from work. What do you notice about how being in nature makes you feel?

Have a go

we gain the time to fully experience and appreciate our sensations and actions.

### Nature does not rush

We can learn a lot from nature – it takes its time yet still gets things done. With the passing of the seasons, first come buds, then flowers, then eventually decay – nature teaches us about the slow, steady, inevitable cycle of life and death that our mindless rushing cannot change. Tuning into the natural world by walking through a park, getting our hands dirty in the garden, or practising mindful movement outdoors allows us to fully appreciate the value and richness of each precious moment in life. Not only that, observing natural as opposed to urban scenes can restore

## Pause right now

Take this opportunity to stop – put the book down straightaway and do nothing. Now take three breaths. What happened?

Have a go

our attentional capacities and improve executive attention,[3] the type of attention we need to train in mindfulness (see page 77).[4]

Taoist philosophy draws heavily on the observation of nature and the *Tao Te Ching* espouses the advantages of doing less:

> 'In the pursuit of Tao, every day something is dropped. Less and less is done. Until non-action is achieved. When nothing is done, nothing is left undone.'
>
> *Tao Te Ching*, Chapter 48

It's not that we need to stop doing things altogether, but rather that we should drop the pushing and striving future-orientation that keeps us out of the present moment. This creates a new spaciousness in the mind, enabling us to think and see more clearly so that we are better able to focus on the things that really matter.

## Coping with external factors

Many factors beyond our control influence how we pace ourselves – not least, the place where we happen to be. I've noticed that life goes at a breakneck speed in São Paulo, Brazil, a city fuelled by caffeine and adrenaline; and that my Londoner's walking speed seemed frantic in laid-back Barbados, where it took me a few days to adjust. But even in the most hectic of cities, there are opportunities to

Spending a few minutes contemplating the unhurried yet inevitable changes of the natural world can offer instant escape from the frenetic pace of modern life.

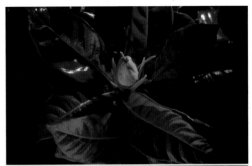
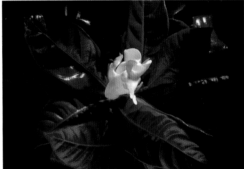
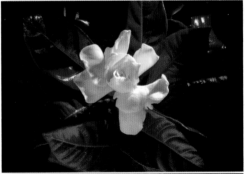
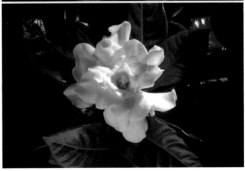

## Control centre for internal pacing

Tucked under the base of your skull, your cerebellum provides your brain with information about timing and the sequence of events. This timing information is not only important for the smooth execution of physical movements, but also for planning and ordering your thoughts and speech. If the cerebellum is damaged, the person will experience a range of difficulties across their cognitive, emotional and motor functions. This suggests there may be common processes underlying brain function which are controlled by common neural structures. The way the timing information is used may be different depending on the task (moving your arm, for example, or planning your next holiday), but always requires temporal ordering and the engagement of the cerebellum. As we will see later (see pages 48–9), when working with processes that cut across different domains (motor, cognitive, emotional), there is a possibility to train in one domain (in this book, the motor domain) to facilitate development in the other domains (cognitive and emotional). For this reason training with the body and movement can allow us to reap benefits in the realms of thinking and feeling.

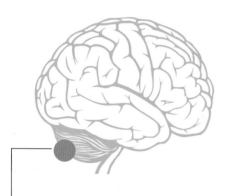

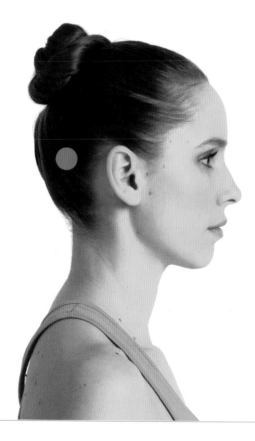

The red dots show the position of the cerebellum, which controls your brain's understanding of timing and the sequencing of events.[5]

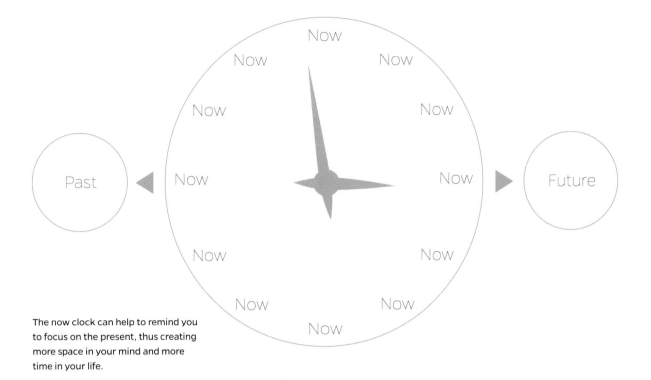

The now clock can help to remind you to focus on the present, thus creating more space in your mind and more time in your life.

connect with nature and set your own pace. In London I find that taking time out in a quiet area of greenery is a really helpful way to slow down.

Noticing the influence of external factors on the way you pace yourself can support you as you develop your mindfulness practice. Ultimately, try to become aware of your internal speedometer, so that you can choose your own pace, from the inside, wherever you are.

## Using your body to access 'now'

Physically slowing down your body, even by just walking more slowly, is a great way to start exploring your mental and physical pacing habits.

I use a picture of the now clock (see above) to help me to remember that each passing second is an opportunity to be present. These now moments are not just seconds ticking down before some impending future event, they *are* our life; they are all we really have. Those who have suffered sudden illness or a near-death experience know exactly what it feels like to value the moment that is now. With continued mindfulness practice, as you learn to live more and more in the present, your now moments can expand, creating more space in your mind and more time in your life for the people and things that matter to you.

As you zip through your life, all sorts of sensations, sights and emotions that lie on the fringes of your awareness pass by you without your full attention. Physically stopping the body in a traditional seated meditation practice is one way to observe what unfolds in the mental space; mindful movement is another.

# Let's practise:
# swimming backward

So many of us hold tension in our shoulders and neck and the surrounding muscles. This is a wonderful exercise to help release this tension. Completed slowly and mindfully, the movement also helps us to stay present and observe our experience as it unfolds over time. Practise the exercise for 5 to 10 minutes, sitting or standing, indoors or outside.

① First, familiarize yourself with the movement. Adopt the tai chi standing posture, feet facing forward, knees slightly bent, pelvis tucked under slightly and with an alert but relaxed posture through your torso. Let your hands rest by your sides, palms down and fingers pointing forward. Alternatively, sit in an alert but relaxed upright posture, with enough room to swing your arms.

② Begin by bringing up your non-dominant arm (so, your left arm if you are right-handed).

③ Lift your non-dominant arm above your head.

④ And bring it down behind you to complete the circle. Repeat steps 1–4 at a pace that comes naturally to you to get the hang of the movement.

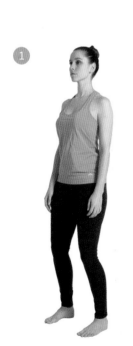

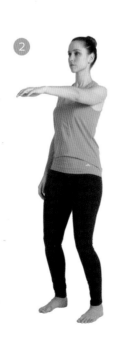

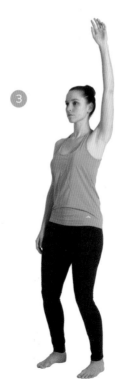

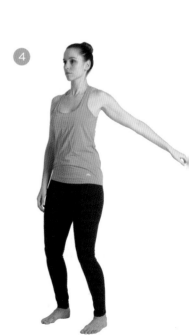

(5) Now repeat the movement more slowly. Bring one arm up, raising it slowly with full relaxation and attention.

(6) Reach up at the apex of the movement, feeling a slight extension in your arm and rotating your palm outward as you do so.

(7) Continue the circular movement as you rotate your shoulder and bring your arm down behind you, as if you were slowly swimming backward.

(8) After a few circles, switch to your other arm. Then return to your non-dominant arm and repeat the movement a few times, reducing your arm speed even further. Repeat with your other arm. Try to keep your movements smooth and continuous, checking in to see if there is a chance to soften or release tension anywhere in your body. Periodically, check that the lower half of your body and your face are as relaxed as possible.

5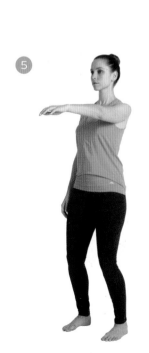

6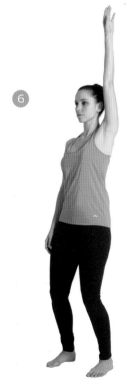

7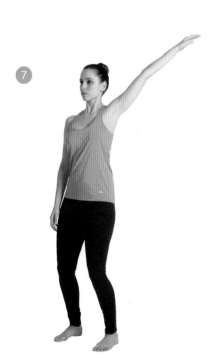

# swimming backward
# (continued)

(9) Now that you've got the gist of the movement, let's use mindfulness principles to really explore the sensations. Starting with your non-dominant arm, make the swimming backward movement, noticing any sensations in your shoulder – particularly the effort you need to make to begin and execute the turn in your arm. Focus only on your hand and wrist for a few strokes. Feel the air against your hand as it sweeps around. Can you feel any regions of tension or relaxation in your wrist or hand as they move? Rotate your wrist and play with the orientation of your hand throughout the turn of your arm – how do the sensations change as the positions of your hand change?

(10) Focus your mind on the timing of movements as each of your muscles engages in order to complete the arm movement. What do you notice now ... now ... and now?

(11) At the moment at which your fingers point to the sky, slowly reach higher – as if you are trying to grab fruit from the branch of a tree just out of reach. Stay alert to the sensations in your shoulder socket. How does this stretch affect your ability to make the backward swimming movement?

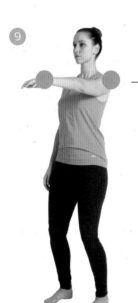

As you swim backward, focus on the sensations in your shoulder, and then in your hand and wrist.

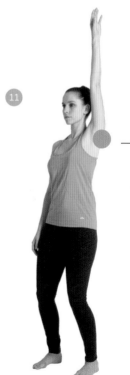

As you reach up, focus on the sensations in your shoulder socket.

⑫ Return your attention to the whole backward swimming movement of your arm. Explore moments of effort and ease throughout. Are there places where you're putting in more effort than you really need to? Is there any point in the movement at which you could exert less, or move with more ease?

⑬ Widen your focus beyond just your arm – what sensations can you notice in your back? Your spine? Your neck?

⑭ Slow your movement down to a stop and, as you do so, notice the transition between movement

and stillness. Give yourself at least 2 or 3 minutes to experience the change in sensation from one to the other. How does the arm that has stopped moving feel different to the arm that has been still?

⑮ Repeat steps 9–14 with your other (stronger) arm. Many people are strongly right- or left-handed, so pay particular attention to any differences in the sensations you feel in your stronger side.

13

Widening your area of focus, be alert to the sensations in your back, your spine and your neck.

Be curious

Now try this ...

○ Lightly touch your moving shoulder with the fingertips of your other hand. Notice the feeling of movement through your fingertips. This feeds another layer of sensation to the brain.

○ Try moving your arm at different speeds. You can work up to a vigorous movement, allowing your arm to swing freely, driving the motion from your waist and keeping your legs firm. Swing your arm round at this speed for ten rotations and then come to rest and stand mindfully noticing the sensations in your arm, shoulder, neck and back. Hold the pause for as long as possible, filling your mind with any sensations in your arm as they unfold over time.

○ Repeat the exercise, again one arm at a time, but this time using a forward circular movement.

○ Try moving only your shoulder, rather than your whole arm.

## What did you discover?

When I started doing this exercise, I noticed very quickly how one shoulder was stiff and sore compared with the other. Straightaway I switched from carrying my laptop in a shoulder bag to carrying it in a backpack, evenly distributing its weight across my body. As we become more mindful, we listen to the body more closely and are able to respond with appropriate corrective action. What pains or stiffness has this exercise highlighted for you? Many people become more aware of their neck muscles, as well as those in the shoulder.

Think about how the exercise alerts you to the thoughts or emotions that arise in response to pleasant or unpleasant sensations in your body. Did any parts of the movement feel especially good to you? Perhaps these were the moments when it was easy to go slow and stay 'curious' (as if observing sensations through the eyes of a child)? Were there moments that felt uncomfortable? Were there moments when you went a bit too fast and it was harder to remain curious?

To be truly mindful, you need to have the same levels of curiosity for *all* your experiences, whether they are pleasant, unpleasant or neutral. Practising mindful movement in this way can help us to see more clearly when we lose curiosity, particularly in response to unpleasant or neutral (sometimes boring or even absent) bodily sensations.

To be truly mindful, you need to have the same levels of curiosity for *all* your experiences.

## Slow it down

Physically slowing down your body, even just by walking more slowly, is a great way to start exploring your pacing habits, both physical and mental. Try a 'pace audit', reviewing your daily habits and observing when you rush, when you are slow and when you conduct your life at a pace that feels natural, alert and calm. You might discover there are certain times and situations when you rush and that this seems unhelpful. These often include eating, commuting or communicating. Try doing all these more slowly. Doing so will allow you to see how your mind and your body interact in these situations. You will have greater access to the wealth of physical and mental sensations that are related to your current experience, making it much richer.

Try a whole day of pausing (see opposite). Slow down your thoughts and actions as you brush your hair or teeth, and eat your breakfast; do the same as you walk to work or to your bus stop. Throughout the day, consciously pause as you transition from one activity to another, such as between meetings or phone calls. Learn to be mindful of the sensations that pass through you as you slow it all down. With a little practice, pausing will soon become second nature.

You can also use your own sensations as a trigger for slowing down. When you notice a particular emotion in your body – for example, a surge of excitement or anger or a wave of anxiety, delight or empathy – slow down and pause to experience the emotion directly. When you deliberately slow down, becoming more aware of how you pace yourself throughout the day, you'll begin to attune much more to how you think and feel, and to the world around you. You may begin to see how physical and mental sensations unfold in your body over time.

Have a go

## A day of pausing

**On waking**
Pause and bring your mind to your body before you even move from your bed.

**Before you eat breakfast**
Connect to the sensations within your body before you take your first mouthful.

**On your commute**
Step to the side and allow one or two people to board in front of you on your bus or train; if you drive, allow someone to pull out from a junction before you. If you're walking, gesture to someone else to pass before you on the pedestrian crossing.

**On reaching your workplace**
Pause as you step over the threshold of your workplace, leaving your journey at the door. Enter your new space fully engaged.

**When your phone rings**
Pause – don't answer straightaway. Allow three full rings before you pick up.

**On receiving an email**
Pause – can you resist the urge to look at the content straightaway? Pause again before replying, and again before you press 'send'.

**When you notice a feeling**
Pause – stop what you're doing and fully explore the sensations in your body.

# Mindful movement and the passage of time

By observing the unfolding of your movements and sensations, you can train yourself to stop negative emotions in their tracks.

Practising mindful movement trains your brain to become more sensitive to the sequencing of mental and physical events in your body. For example, try mindful walking and notice how it takes you moment by moment through time: 'First I shift my weight onto the right foot, then I lift the left foot, then I swing the left leg, then the left foot touches the floor ...' and so on. The more we practise walking mindfully, the more we engage fully with every moment.

We can also experience bodily sensations on a moment-by-moment basis, and these too give us a vehicle through which we can watch time unfold (for example, first the sensations of sitting in the seat of a chair, then of your back against the chair, then the tactile sensations of your clothing, then those of the temperature of your skin and so on). If you can practise this level of mindfulness regularly, you may be able to develop the ability to distinguish

Every movement can be broken down into smaller stages. This is the midnight sun, its passage caught by time-lapse photography in Alaska at summer solstice.

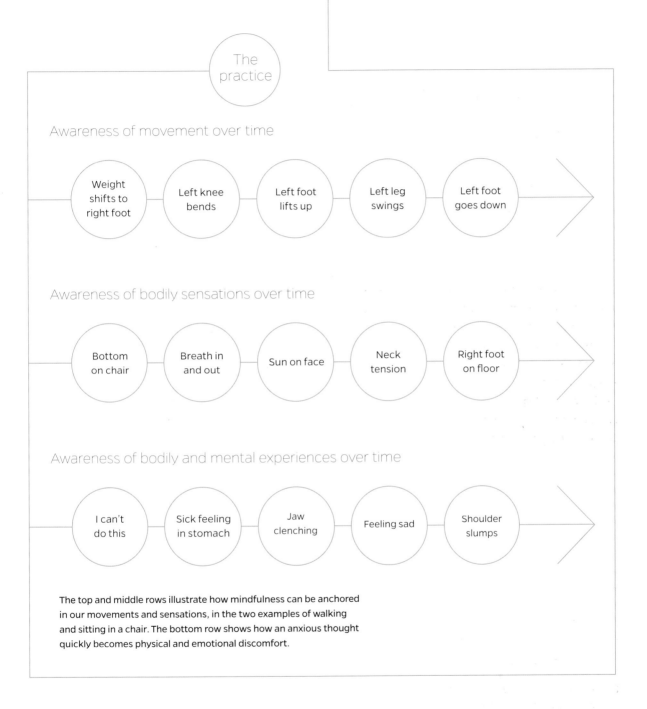

The practice

Awareness of movement over time

Weight shifts to right foot → Left knee bends → Left foot lifts up → Left leg swings → Left foot goes down

Awareness of bodily sensations over time

Bottom on chair → Breath in and out → Sun on face → Neck tension → Right foot on floor

Awareness of bodily and mental experiences over time

I can't do this → Sick feeling in stomach → Jaw clenching → Feeling sad → Shoulder slumps

The top and middle rows illustrate how mindfulness can be anchored in our movements and sensations, in the two examples of walking and sitting in a chair. The bottom row shows how an anxious thought quickly becomes physical and emotional discomfort.

increasingly fine detail in the timing and sequencing of your mental events. And once you can do this, you'll be in a position to catch unwanted habitual negative thoughts earlier in their development, so that you can eventually eliminate them altogether from your thinking.

# Let's practise: bodily movements and breathing

This exercise helps you to notice the passage of time by observing how your breathing triggers a sequence of sensations in your body. You can practise the exercise anywhere and at any time, but it is most effective when you're sitting or lying down and if you can practise for 5–10 minutes.

① Focus on your torso (the region between your neck and tummy). Tune into any sensations you feel moving through you in this area.

② Breathe in, and out, at whatever pace your breath is right now. Follow any sensations and movements in your torso. Where do you feel your breath as you breathe in – in the first instant, in the second and so on? What movement do you feel and where, moment by moment, as the breath moves through you? Close your eyes and connect to the movements and sensations in your body.

③ Place one hand on your chest and one on your tummy. Continue to breathe at whatever pace is natural to you. The breath may slow but it doesn't have to do so for this or any other exercise; rather it should be smooth and continuous. Move your awareness from the movement of your breath to the movement of your hands as they rise and fall. Now, focus on the movement of your breath through the front and back of your torso.

## A note about breathing

In tai chi, there is little instruction about the breath, other than for it to be silent, smooth and continuous. Training the breath in this way means it will naturally adjust to your exertion level and sync to your movements, without you having to do any special breathing sequences.

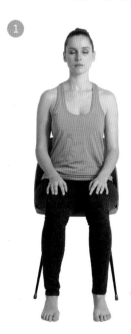

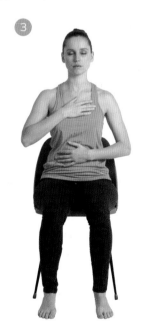

# Learning to inhibit your movements

Training in mindful movement of your body can help you to learn how to regulate your thoughts and emotions.

A s you may have discovered in the Swimming Backward exercise (see pages 36–9), moving slowly and mindfully is hard – and takes effort. In 2001 I was part of a team that published a paper mapping the neural networks we use to achieve motor inhibition (in lay terms, the pathways in the brain we use to slow down or stop our movement). In that paper we wrote that 'Every behavioural, cognitive, or motor act requires a finely tuned balance between initiatory and inhibitory processes to provide appropriate preparation, initiation, on-line control, and timely inhibition of this act.'[6]

Your motor system is the part of the nervous system that controls your movements. You use inhibitory processes when you need to change your movement (for example, when you need to walk around an obstacle) and also when you need to stop a movement you've already begun (when you slow down). Inhibitory processes happen along pathways in the right hemisphere of the brain, including those in the inferior and medial frontal cortex and parietal lobes. When you make a slow movement, activation in these regions changes the motor programme, pulling on the breaks and slowing it down.

We know from studies of tai chi practice in the elderly that consistent use of these pathways improves a person's ability to activate motor inhibition when necessary – and for older adults this has meant fewer trips and falls.[7] The person is simply better able to adapt the motor programme whenever they encounter an obstacle.

But it's not just our motor system that has related inhibition pathways. Other parts of the brain are responsible for cognitive inhibition and emotional inhibition.[8] You'll use cognitive inhibition when you're working in a busy office and have to pull your mind away from the distraction of colleagues chatting or machinery whirring around you. You'll use emotional inhibition when you notice you're starting to feel overwhelmed and want to hold it in – think about the times you've pulled back (even if it's only briefly) when you've felt like bursting into tears or screaming.

The ability to inhibit behaviours, thoughts and emotions is vital to our ability to function in the world. When it is compromised (for example, in those who suffer from Attention Deficit Hyperactivity Disorder) problems with social functioning occur. However, excessive inhibition of emotions is also not good for you – if you suppress your negative feelings such as anger or guilt, you are at higher risk of depression.[9]

Mindfulness can train you how to strike a skilful balance. Put simply, mindfulness teaches us not to inhibit or stop the emotions altogether, but to use our emotional inhibition mechanisms *sparingly* and appropriately, so that we can better regulate our emotional states and lead happier, healthier lives.

BMT exercises predominantly train your motor inhibition, but links within the brain mean that they also give you some extra 'oomph' to call on when you need to pull back your thought processes or your emotions.[10]

## Motor and cognitive inhibition in daily life

Have you ever sent an email that you wished you could take back? Training in mindful movement encourages you to sense, observe and inhibit the move toward 'send' and in that momentary space, allow you to listen to your gut feeling ('not a good idea') and stop sending altogether, or to read through what you've written one more time to ensure everything you've said is exactly as it needs to be.

In a study I conducted with colleagues in Brazil, lay meditators demonstrated an ability to observe, from the inside, their imminent execution of a movement and pull it back.[11] This enhanced the appropriateness and accuracy of their actions.

Have you ever had to 'bite your tongue'? If so, it's likely you were inhibiting in all three domains of behaviour, thoughts and emotions, engaging the important right ventrolateral region of the brain (see illustration, below). You may often strongly feel the physical sense of the motor command to speak unfolding around your mouth. Although you don't literally bite your tongue, you do stop your lips from moving! You can, then, with practice, see thoughts and actions arising and deliberately pull back. Pausing before speaking allows you to observe both the cognitive (planning the words) and motor (speech production) inhibition networks in action. Depending on the situation, there might also be an emotional component. Try the exercise opposite.

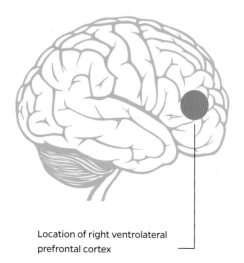

Location of right ventrolateral prefrontal cortex

## Key brain region for inhibition

Inhibitory processes happen predominantly along pathways in the right hemisphere of the brain, including the inferior and medial frontal cortex and the parietal lobes. A recent survey points to the right ventrolateral prefontal cortex as a key region involved in inhibition, cutting across the domains of motor, thinking and emotion regulation.[12]

## Pause before speaking

Add a 3-second pause the next time you speak
to or respond to someone.

○ What did you observe?

○ Were you able to notice the muscles around your
mouth preparing for speech?

○ In what ways could you sense that your decision
to pause inhibited the movement of your mouth?

○ What did you observe in your mind during
that pause?

Try speaking 10 per cent less tomorrow. Then 20 per
cent less the following day. Then 50 per cent less the
day after that. Observe what you're doing to reduce
the amount you're talking.

Pulling back and pausing means that you can
respond rather than react. If you create a habit of
pausing, you will give yourself a choice in those split
seconds during which you might otherwise react
emotionally. Perhaps you were going to shout at a
family member, but pulling back means that you can
respond calmly; perhaps you were going to berate
the assistant in your local store, but instead you can
choose to ask for help from another assistant, or to
leave and shop elsewhere. Your pause creates space
and within that created space time for a more skilful
response. Becoming good at pausing before speaking
takes practice, however, especially if your emotions
are running high, but keep practising and you *will* find
it easier in time.

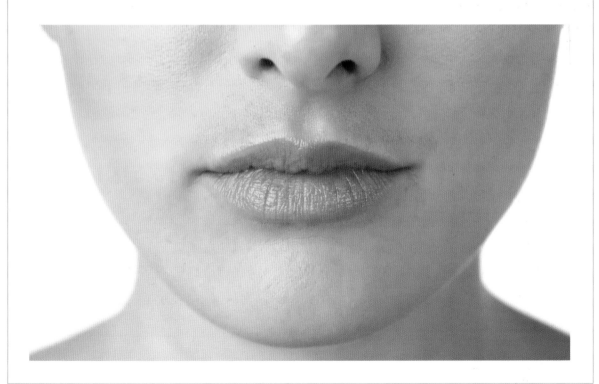

# Touching the present

We can reflect on what we have done and also project our mind into the future, but the body is a relatively simple machine. We might remember sitting on a hard chair but we can't recapture the actual sensations. The body binds us to the *present* moment.

In any moment your body sends millions of signals to your brain, providing detailed information about everything from movement and digestion to temperature regulation and your emotional state. Most of this information is outside our awareness – we don't notice it happening – unless, that is, we choose to look carefully, with mindfulness.

Attending to the raw sensations of the body on a moment-by-moment basis means turning your mind's eye to the activity going on in the somatosensory cortex of your brain. It's this area and the adjacent motor cortex that are active when we move our bodies. These areas receive and relay messages from and to the body, providing data about the changing sensations as we move. Focusing on these sensations may allow us to access via awareness the rawest form of data about our bodies. For the execution of movement, neurons in the somatosensory cortex communicate with those in the adjacent primary motor cortex and the supplementary motor areas. By attending to the moving body, you can tap into the sensations represented and processed across multiple brain regions.

Our task in mindfulness training, particularly when we go deep into the body, is to know the difference between *thinking* about, say, the hand (facts, images, memories and so on) and really *feeling* the raw sensations of the hand as they enter the brain.

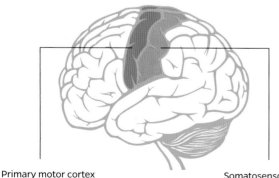

Primary motor cortex                    Somatosensory cortex

## The brain's command centre

The somatosensory cortex interprets messages from, say, your hand, as information travels up your spinal column. It then communicates with the motor areas, to generate movement.

Your brain is good at short-cutting true sensation in this way. You may have noticed when you tried to connect to the raw sensations of your body (see exercise on pages 36–9) that you experience an image (of your hand, for example) or a thought about it – a label related to the movement you're making, but not the movement itself. Remember that the aim is to observe the actual movement moment by moment through the neural activity in the somatosensory cortex. If you're concentrating on what your hand looks like, you have switched to observing activity in other brain regions.

Try the next exercise (right) to experience the different levels on which your mind perceives your body. The exercises on pages 50–51 are designed to help you develop a new habit of 'dropping into your body' – deepening your awareness of your physical sensations. Dropping into the body and moving it a bit is essential for people who spend long hours sitting, as it gives the body a chance to stretch, and brings us out of our thoughts to focus on the present rather than worrying about the future or the past.

## Letting go of labels

Have a go

Pay attention to one hand (it doesn't matter which). Allow your mind to generate images of hands, knowledge about hands, memories of hands. What happens? Now, deliberately drop any images or labels and attend to the raw sensations of your chosen hand. It may help to rest your hand on a surface so that you have something to feel it against.

Now experiment with separating your verbal labelling of your hand from your experience of it. Repeat the word 'hand' in your head but, as you do so, practise letting go of the label itself and instead rest your mind on the raw sensation of your hand.

For every exercise in the book, become aware when you find your mind wandering from raw sensation to images or verbal labels and bring it back into mindful movement. With practice, you'll soon get the hang of staying fully in the moment.

## Progression of raw sensation over time

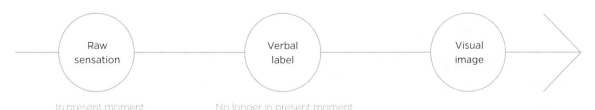

| Raw sensation | Verbal label | Visual image |
|---|---|---|
| In present moment | No longer in present moment | |

When we experience a raw sensation, the mind quickly gives it a verbal label or visual image. Mindfulness training helps us to identify when we have left our present sensations and to return to them as soon as possible.

# Let's practise:
# posture take two

Regular practice of this exercise trains you to stay in your body and in the present moment, as well as improving your posture and body awareness. At first, do it in a quiet environment for 5 to 10 minutes so that you can really notice all the sensations. After practice you can do a shorter version whenever you sit down.

① Find a seated posture that is both alert and relaxed. Place your hands on your lap so that your arms are fully supported. Breathe out and begin to drop your attention into your body, deliberately releasing or pulling back from your busy (thinking) mind into the raw sensations in your bones, muscles and skin. Use your out-breath to help you find the place(s) in your body where you notice the effects of gravity. Observe regions where there is pressure – places where your flesh feels compressed. Be alert to the temperature of the air against your skin, the texture of your clothes and other tactile sensations.

② On the next in-breath, pull in your tummy slightly and feel the elongation of your spine; sense yourself growing tall. Keep your spine alert, then breathe out again, letting the muscles, tendons and flesh around your skeleton release and relax. Be alert to visual imagery and verbal labels, and drop them promptly.

③ Breathe in again and as you breathe out use the exhalation to guide your attention systematically down through your neck and shoulders, chest and torso – breathe out as if you are breathing down through your arms and into your hands in your lap.

④ As you breathe out, use your mind to release any tension in your lower back, letting your muscles drop, bringing your attention down to your hips and pelvis. Notice how your pelvis holds your torso on the chair.

⑤ Bring your attention all the way down to your feet on the floor. Make the sensory input from your body your main priority, greeting sensations with a high degree of curiosity – as if you were experiencing them for the first time, through the eyes of a child. Keep looking, observing, noticing in this moment, now this moment, now this moment ... and the next.

⑥ Observe any sensations in your feet (say, from your socks or shoes). Attend to the left and right foot in turn. If you notice any mental activity, such as planning, judging, analysing, don't resist, just go with it, then gently pull back or inhibit the chain of thought and re-establish bodily sensations as your main focus.

Have a go

## Focusing on posture

There are many moments in daily life when you can bring your body fully into mind. Try it when you are:

○ waiting for the bus/train/photocopier/kettle;

○ typing or searching the Internet;

○ making a telephone call;

○ eating/cooking/shopping.

# Let's practise:
# right here right now

This exercise is a great antidote to a busy, restless mind. You can practise it anywhere – in the loo, at your desk, in the supermarket queue, even in the middle of the night when you can't sleep. Use it in neutral moments, positive moments and negative moments. Explore all the possibilities. You can have your eyes opened or closed throughout, and you can systematically work through your body from head to toe, or simply engage with sensations as they arise. With practice, you will notice you gain a greater ability to disengage from mental activity and remain present, using the body as an anchor for your attention. It should take around 5 to 10 minutes.

① Wherever you are, seated or standing, pause, stop and bring your attention to 'right here, right now' directly into the body. What aspects of your body come into your awareness? How do they unfold over time?

② Play around with adding some general labels for the things you notice (hand, breath, ribs, feet, tingling, face and so on) and then drop these labels, focusing fully on the raw sensations themselves. Remember the now clock (see page 35) – keep asking yourself 'What is happening now? And now? And now ...?'

Have a go

## Check in with your body

Try a gentle neck stretch, tipping your head from side to side to bring your ear toward your shoulder on each side. Remember to practise slowly and with full attention to the raw sensations of your body. When I do this exercise in the library or on the bus, I often find that others start to do it around me. A nice ripple effect occurs – when we show we care for our own bodies, we give others around us the permission to care for their bodies, too. Give it a go!

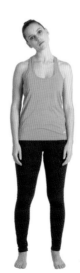
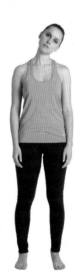

# Mindfulness of your emotions

Although we might think of emotions as non-physical, in fact they ripple throughout our body. For this reason, staying as close as possible to the raw sensations of the body becomes particularly important when we are dealing with high emotion.

A s soon as an emotion rises within us, the brain tends to label it – just as it does sensations. Again, this moves us away from the brain regions that code primary body sensations and into the regions for processing and conceptual understanding.[13] As soon as the labels begin, we are no longer fully present in the experience of the emotion; we are susceptible to the brain's misinterpretations. Think back to a time when an experience caused an emotional reaction. If you labelled that reaction as 'fear', say, it probably became fear before you had an opportunity to really study it. Perhaps it wasn't fear, but excitement? Anger can often be confused with sadness. These are the sorts of trick your mind can play. Alternatively, if your conceptual mind is too quick to label and process your emotions, you could miss out on the direct experience of emotion in your body – you may lose your ability to discern what you are really feeling, diminishing your emotional life.

Pause now and reflect on what 'that really moved me' means to you. For me, it represents the wave of emotion that moves through my body when I have a strong response. It's far from being a conceptual reaction. This sense of emotion felt in the body is activated in a region of the brain called the insula.[14] In many studies, experienced meditators show an increase in insula size, particularly on the brain's right side. This increase is directly correlated to the number of years the person has practised meditation.[15] A larger, more densely connected insula equates to more emotional sensitivity.

Different emotions have different bodily 'signatures'.[16] As the studies into experienced meditators show us, remaining connected to the raw sensations in your body will help you to experience a dramatic increase in your emotional intelligence. You can develop confidence in your ability to sit with difficult emotions, and you'll become better able to detect changes in your emotional state, spotting them earlier and responding in the most appropriate way before the emotions overwhelm you.

Remaining in the moment, fully experiencing your emotions in the body and observing how they unfold over time takes courage when your emotions are intense. Regular mindfulness practice will make this experience possible and help you manage it. Use the exercise on page 54 to guide you.

As a surfer rides a wave with grace and courage, so we can train ourselves to flow with our emotions as they peak and subside.

## Overcoming
## emotional avoidance

Some people find it extremely difficult to attend to emotions in the body. Avoidance – allowing emotions to pass through awareness as quickly as possible without giving them proper attention – probably worked for that person at one time in their life, but when avoidance becomes deeply ingrained and habitual, the fear of facing certain emotions can feel so overwhelming that avoidance seems to be the only option.

In my clinical practice, I use BMT to help clients to stay with and be curious about the movement of strong emotions through their bodies. This encourages them to become aware of the onset of an emotion, its full force and its gradual fading away.

We often use the metaphor that the life of an emotion is like a wave. We ask ourselves if we can surf the wave of emotion, rather than trying to suppress it, fight it or interfere with it. The time it takes for the emotion to arise and fade away is much shorter than we think as long as we stay with it and allow it to diminish on its own, rather than trying to avoid it.

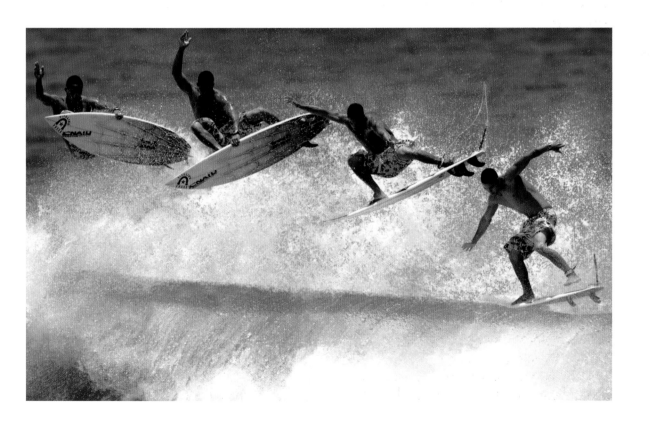

# Let's practise:
# pausing in the thick of it

The mild to moderate stressors in life provide a good starting point for practising mindfulness of the emotions in the body. Road rage, commute rage, queue-jumping, technology failure – to name just a few – are all situations in which we can start to get familiar with how the body feels the emotions of frustration, irritation and anger.

(1) As soon as you feel an emotion rising within you (often when something happens that is unwanted or unpleasant), pause, focus your mind directly on your torso, and just watch ... and watch ... observe how your bodily sensations rise and fade away. Be alert to the 'stories' (the labels and predictions) your mind wants to give each emotion. Each time you see your mind trying to take control in this way, pull back and stay directly with your raw bodily sensations, experiencing them unfold over time – stay present.

(2) Once you are comfortable and confident with this technique, try to use it in situations that have a higher emotional charge. For example, use it when you have to have a meeting with a difficult person at work. Notice the feelings in your body in anticipation of the event, as well as those that arise during the interaction itself.

---

Have a go

## Mood and movement

Beginning to notice how emotions move through the body and the effect that they have on our physical being is a great way to build emotional awareness and emotional intelligence. Nuances in our movements can tell us a lot about how we are feeling in a given situation.[17] Take every chance you are offered to observe how bodily movements and sensations are impacted as you go about your daily life. Pay particular attention to those moments when you are:

(1) becoming upset, worried or anxious about something;

(2) engaging in an activity that is pleasurable.

Notice if your bodily movements speed up or slow down and how your muscle tone changes. What happens to your level of co-ordination and physical precision?

Observe how others are moving and see if you can evaluate their mood. An American research laboratory called Bio Motion Lab have created an online experiment that explores our ability to infer mood from movement.[18]

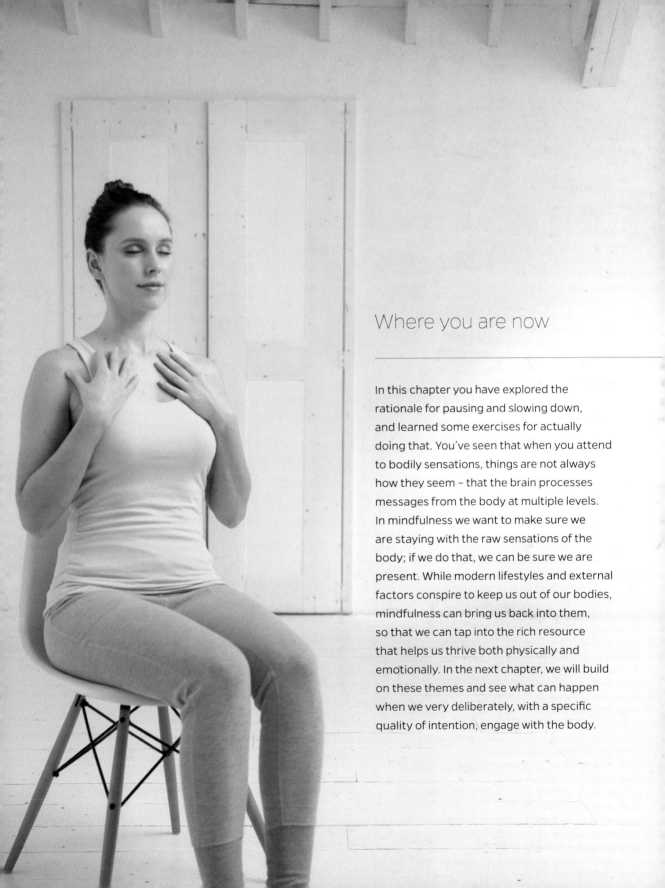

## Where you are now

In this chapter you have explored the
rationale for pausing and slowing down,
and learned some exercises for actually
doing that. You've seen that when you attend
to bodily sensations, things are not always
how they seem – that the brain processes
messages from the body at multiple levels.
In mindfulness we want to make sure we
are staying with the raw sensations of the
body; if we do that, we can be sure we are
present. While modern lifestyles and external
factors conspire to keep us out of our bodies,
mindfulness can bring us back into them,
so that we can tap into the rich resource
that helps us thrive both physically and
emotionally. In the next chapter, we will build
on these themes and see what can happen
when we very deliberately, with a specific
quality of intention, engage with the body.

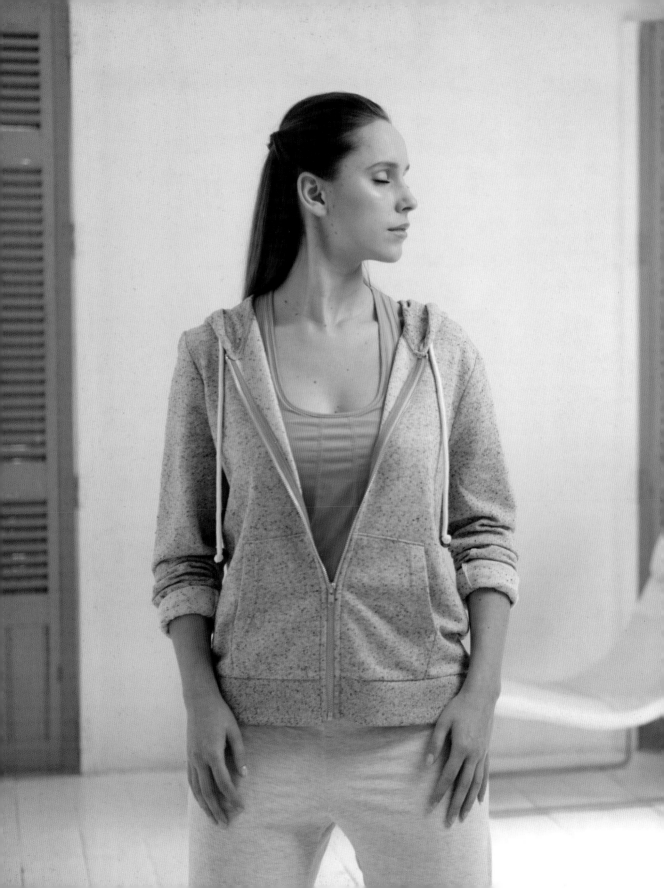

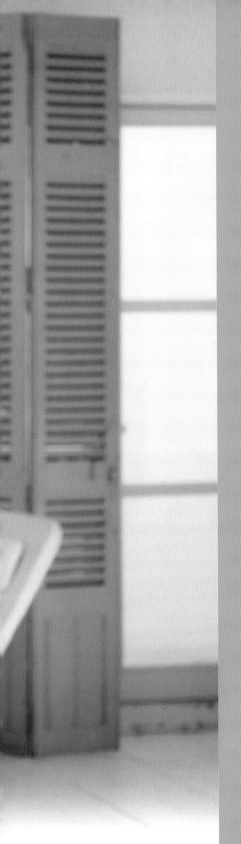
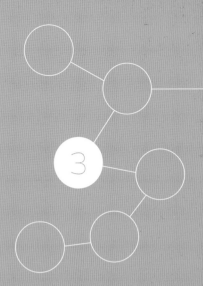

# Intention

The previous chapter gave you an opportunity
to observe more of your internal and external
experience. Pausing can help you to see what
lies behind your actions and reactions – it is the
window to your intentions. In this chapter I'll show
you how to set your intention by thinking about
how you want to think, speak, move or act, and
how to be mindful as you go about fulfilling your
intention. We'll look at how an intention is different
from a goal, and how your intention has a ripple
effect all around you. We'll use BMT exercises to
explore the links between your intention and your
movement, so that you can develop a deeper
understanding of your wider intentions in life,
and of the intentions of others.

# What is intention?

Intention is part of decision-making, keeping us on our path. In tai chi it is a type of mental activity that is both purposeful and relaxed. It is also a key part of mindfulness; the point to which we return again and again.

B roadly speaking the word 'intention' refers to a plan, a purpose, an aim or a commitment to do something. Interestingly, in Buddhism, the Pali interpretation of the word *sati* (which is loosely translated as mindfulness), uses the phrase 'intentness of mind' to reflect a firm commitment to engage with mental experience without distraction. Intentions are often classified as 'good' or 'bad' and are assumed to have some decision behind them. Deliberately setting intentions makes it easier to stay on track with a plan, helping us to notice more quickly when we deviate. This occurs at the micro level – moment by moment returning to our intention

Have a go

## Tap in to your intention

Take a moment to recall your intention when you selected this book, perhaps asking:

○ What was I hoping to achieve by reading this book?

○ What led me to select a book about mindful movement?

○ Why am I interested in mindfulness?

As you do so, what do you notice in your body? What do you notice in your mind?

Reflect on this

## Intention or goal?

Setting intentions is very different from setting goals. Consider the difference between the words *intention* and *goal*. First, drop the word *goal* into your mind and then observe any words, images, thoughts or bodily sensations that arise. Repeat the word a few times. Now do the same for *intention*. The experience of this exercise really surprised me, so much so that I now try to work exclusively with intentions in every realm of my life. Goals have a rigid, external feel. They are 'out there' and we either achieve or don't achieve them. If we apparently fail to reach our goals, we may be hard on ourselves and discard the successes we make en route. Intention, on the other hand, has a softer, more flexible, dynamic feel. It has scope for modification and updating. Intention connects us to the stages of the journey, not just to a fixed end point, so success and failure are immeasurable – there's only the journey itself.

during mindfulness meditation practice; and at the macro level, in the more far-reaching plans we have for our lives.

## Intention and tai chi

Tai chi teachers often use the phrase 'Where the mind goes, the *chi* flows' and the Tai Chi Classics tell us that *qi* (energy) follows *yi* (intention).[1] Intention is the 'alert but relaxed' movement of consciousness into the body and it creates a path along which our mental energy flows. Interestingly, the Latin word *intentus*, from which we get the English intention, means 'an extending'. At the more advanced level, the concept of *yi* is intention that travels out beyond our physical body.

In tai chi, practitioners use 'push hands' and pair work to develop sensitivity to intentions – their own and those of their opponents. Humans have an innate ability to read each other's intentions,[2] a skill that evolved to allow us to live harmoniously in large social groups. From an evolutionary perspective, our brains needed to develop a way to determine quickly whether something moving rapidly toward us had a good intention or a bad one – whether it wanted to offer friendship or love, or to devour us! Mindful movement taps into this primal ability, allowing us to hone our innate social skills.

## Intention in mindfulness theory

In modern mindfulness theory,[3] three separate but interconnecting concepts – intention, attention and attitude (IAA) – together create the experience we call 'mindfulness'.

When practising mindfulness we move between these three processes. We intend (*intention*) to pay *attention* to our mental and physical experiences in

Have a go

## Walking intention

The next time you walk down a busy street, deliberately project your intention in front of you. Fix your gaze on your path and maintain an awareness of your body and posture.

A student told me he does this while travelling through the busy London Underground system at rush hour. What has surprised him most is the ease with which he can move through this busy environment. It seems as if people move out of his way, as if he creates a river of *qi* that people avoid stepping through. He experienced the human ability to read intention in action (see page 68).

a kind and non-judgmental way (*attitude*). One second later our mind wanders and we realize we are no longer doing what was intended. We try our best not to judge (*attitude*), and then renew or refresh our *intention* to pay *attention*. This cycle repeats many times, perhaps even hundreds of times, during a mindfulness practice.

IAA provides me with my daily guiding principle – it reminds me to check that I am living as mindfully as possible. Try to get into the habit of asking yourself, 'What is my intention with this act?', 'What will distract my attention and pull me off course?' and 'Am I acting with kindness?' about every task you perform.

## Bringing intention into awareness

When we make intentions explicit – when we bring them into our awareness – we create a template for our intended experience in our minds. It's like telling

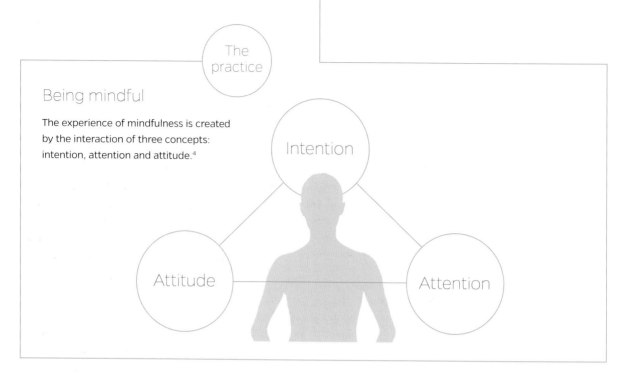

## Being mindful

The experience of mindfulness is created by the interaction of three concepts: intention, attention and attitude.[4]

Intention

Attitude

Attention

the brain over and over again, 'This is what I want to do; this is what I want to do.' Then, when we go off track (as inevitably we will) and deviate from the template, we notice more quickly what is happening and so can more quickly bring ourselves back to our intention.

### The yin and yang of going off track

If we understand what it means to be 'on track', following the path of our intention, we must by definition understand when we go 'off track', too. This principle of opposites informing each other is described in the ying and yang theory that underpins tai chi and the Taoist philosophy.

> 'When you move upward, the mind must
> be aware of down; when moving forward,
> the mind also thinks of moving back.'
> *Tai Chi Classics*

It's the same in mindfulness practice:

○ Learning INattention helps us to hone our ability to pay attention.

○ Learning about mindLESS moments (when our minds wander) informs our understanding of what it means to be mindFUL.

○ Learning when we feel UNease, informs us about what it means to be at ease.

○ Seeing when we are UNkind to ourselves, increases our ability to be kind and compassionate.

When you are aware of inattention, mindlessness or unease, you have an opportunity to embrace and love even your most uncertain moments, as these are actually your greatest learning opportunities.

# Let's practise:
# mindfulness of the breath

In this exercise you will do the same practice twice but with different levels of intentionality. Allow 5 minutes for each breathing practice (10 minutes altogether). You can practise this exercise anywhere and anytime, but will achieve the best results if you are in a quiet environment. It might help to set an alarm for each 5 minutes so that you don't become preoccupied with watching the time.

① Attend to your breath for 5 minutes – do nothing other than focus on it as you breathe in and out in a regular pattern. What did you notice?

② Now do it again, but this time start by stating your intention that your breath will be the main and only focus of your attention. State this intention

mentally or out loud, perhaps with the thought, 'I will now attend to the breath', and then really stick to it. This means that any time you notice you are not attending to the breath, you might quickly label this mental experience 'not breath' and then drop it as fast as possible and return your attention to the breath. As soon as you notice your mind wandering, repeat the phrase to renew your intention.

What did you notice? Was there any difference in your ability to stay with the practice? Try explicit intention setting as you do the other practices in this book.

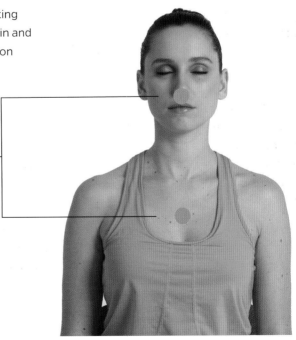

Focus on your breath as it enters your body through your mouth or nose, fills your lungs and is then expelled from your body, completing the cycle.

# How intentions change over time

As you settle into a regular mindfulness practice – whether seated or moving – you will naturally adapt your initial intentions.

A s you settle into a regular mindfulness practice – whether seated or moving – your intentions will naturally change over time. For example, you may have begun with fixed intentions to eliminate all negative experiences from your life, but find that this morphs into a new intention to engage with all experience – even when it is negative. (Practitioners who are coping with depression often begin with the intention to remove their low moods altogether, but soon understand that it's kinder to the self to instead set the intention to observe periods of low mood with more compassion.)

Many studies show that it is this transformed intention to become more compassionate toward ourselves that seems to underpin many of the positive effects of regular mindfulness training.[5]

## Setting intentions during transitional phases

**The practice**

When you transition from one phase of your life to the next, you may find it helpful to engage explicitly with your intentions. This is intentionality at the macro level. If you are changing jobs or relationships, or if perhaps you are about to become a parent or grandparent, or experience what it's like when your last child leaves home, your underlying intentions for your life and self are likely to shift. Remember that setting intentions gives you a flexible framework for life, and that revising your intentions and setting new ones when you are at life's crossroads will guide your future behaviour, helping you to stay fully present in your life. Updating intentions helps you to keep sight of what is really important to you at this period of your life.

# Let's practise:
# dropping the pebble

This 10-minute exercise helps you to explore your intention, expanding on the technique introduced in 'Reflect on This' on page 58. It is called 'Dropping the Pebble' (or, just the 'Pebble') because it encourages you to observe any ripple effect in your body and mind when you drop a question about your intention into your awareness, as if you were letting a pebble fall into water. The more you practise this exercise, the deeper you will be able to connect with those emotions and thoughts that lie outside your awareness. You can practise the exercise any time you have some quiet space to focus.

I use the Pebble exercise all the time – before meetings or client therapy sessions, or before embarking on projects or teaching a mindfulness workshop. I never judge what comes up in my responses; I just experience a deep desire to understand more about what really drives my behaviour. Revisit the Pebble exercise as you progress through the book. By practising repeatedly, you will develop a helpful habit of quickly checking in with your intentions in any situation.

Furthermore, developing your skill at reading your body and mind in relation to your intentions will dramatically increase your chances of staying on track in all areas of your life, from your career to your relationships to your spiritual endeavours. The Pebble exercise is particularly helpful if you are facing a decision that is causing you some uncertainty, confusion or unease, especially during times of transition, as it helps to connect you to your 'gut feeling'.

① Settle into a posture that feels comfortable and presents your body in an alert yet relaxed state. Keep your attention primarily focused on your torso.

② Drop a question into your mind, as if dropping a pebble into a pond, perhaps asking 'What is my intention with BMT?' or 'Why am I practising mindfulness?' Observe any ripples or sensations in your body or mind.

③ Be patient – watch, observing your thoughts, images or bodily sensations as they arise. Resist any urge to analyse or rationalize your answers. Drop the question three times. Each time, wait and observe any response, particularly from your body.

④ Consider the strength or absence of bodily reaction or the presence or absence of mental clarity as you practise this exercise. Does anything about them surprise you? Was the first response the same as or different to your response the second or third time you asked your question?

The Pebble is particularly helpful if you are facing a decision that is causing you some uncertainty, confusion or unease.

# Intention and the brain

Early brain patterns of our motor action form in the brain, representing our intention to move or act. Neuroscientific techniques allow us to observe these signals before we are subjectively aware of them.

B ringing an explicit attentional focus to the intention to move changes the blood flow in these brain regions. In this way, we can be alert to what happens just before we do something, helping us to choose rather than simply react.

Neuroscience research tells us that the brain codes our intention to move some 500 to 2,000 milliseconds before we are actually conscious of the movement.[6] With the intention set before the movement happens, we are able to know when the movement is *not* going as intended. That is, we can quickly deduce when we have gone off track. A similar process happens when we lay out our intention to pay attention to the breath (the brain will alert us more quickly to those 'non-breath' moments), and when we set intentions for our broader lives (alerting us when we are moving away from what is important to us). The neural underpinnings of these latter processes are less well understood. However, in the motor system we can see clearly how this works, with the intention to move preceding commands to move and the subsequent experience of moving our body.

Consider the movement required to pick up a glass of water. Before we move, this preconscious neural activity in the brain creates a type of template of what might be expected in the motor programme to pick up a glass. This template is derived from memories of previous experiences of picking up glasses and collates all the information needed to achieve this goal (such as likely weight and texture of the glass, amount of force and grip needed, the movement to the mouth that has to be made). The brain creates a 'best guess' of the expected sensory consequences of the movement.[7]

When you begin to fulfil your intention to pick up a glass, your movements transmit sensory feedback to the brain, which the brain compares to its original template. If there is a match, the movement has been successful; if there is a mismatch, different brain regions kick in to help you resolve the discrepancy and perhaps change the intended movement. Conscious awareness at this point allows you to revisit your intentions, examine the situation and generate a solution.

Conscious awareness allows you to revisit your intentions, examine the situation and generate a solution.

## How intention unfolds in the brain

The diagrams below show how different parts of your brain generate this intention template prior to the actual execution of the movement.[8] Neural activity spreads from the front to the back of your brain. First, the frontal lobes make the decision to move. Next, the pre-supplementary motor area engages, and starts coding for the anticipated sequence and timing of the movement. The motor cortex makes the final preparations and the command to move is sent down the spinal cord to activate muscles and execute the movement itself. At this point you might be aware of the actual sensory consequences of your moving body coming into the brain.

The pre-supplementary motor area (pre-SMA) of the brain helps to prepare and execute movement – and it is also the brain region that lays down the intention to move. Mindful engagement with the movements of the body trains us to become familiar with this neural activity.

## How mindfulness intervenes in the process

When we practise mindfulness, we place an explicit focus on our decision to move, the unfolding intention and the actual execution of the action. We want to come closer and closer to the origin of the movement – the decision to move – and then watch it unfold over time. Rather then just being aware of the movement, we become aware of our intention to move. In practice, this is similar to the experience of the Mindfulness of the Breath exercise on page 61. When we move, can we become aware of 'I am about to stand up' or 'I will now turn my head' before we actually do it?

The pre-SMA also has a much broader remit, being involved in the planning and execution of cognitive and emotional processes. When we practise the BMT exercises, we bring mindful attention to the intention to move, but because we are connecting with the pre-SMA, we also tap into the intentions that underpin our thoughts and emotional reactions.

### Intention unfolding in the brain before movement

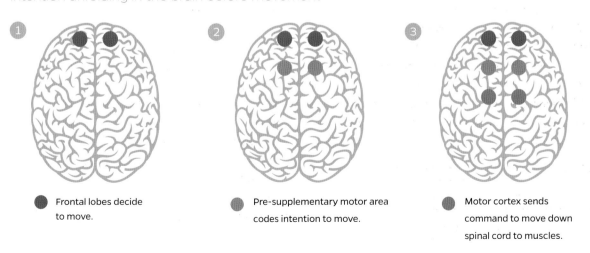

1. Frontal lobes decide to move.

2. Pre-supplementary motor area codes intention to move.

3. Motor cortex sends command to move down spinal cord to muscles.

## Powering up your brain

Turning your 'mind's eye' to the preparatory activity taking place in the pre-SMA boosts its functioning.[9] Pre-SMA neurons begin to fire, which triggers the manufacture and release of neurotransmitters, and increasing blood flow throughout your brain. Generally speaking, the pre-SMA gets a good workout.

Next to the pre-SMA lies the SMA itself, a region of the brain that neuroimaging studies have identified as being influenced by meditation practice.[10] This region connects directly to the motor cortex and the spinal cord and is made of sub-regions that code specifically for action in different body parts. Over time, sustained meditation practice appears to be able to increase the density of neurons in the SMA.

Increased density in the SMA may have some practical benefits, including:

○ greater ability to notice 'urges';

○ greater sensitivity to movement patterns;

○ greater ability to notice when we have gone 'off track', away from our intentions;

○ greater flexibility in our repertoire of movements;

○ greater body awareness in general;

○ greater empathy via the ability to understand the intentions of others.

Have a go

### Swim backward again

Try revisiting the Swimming Backward exercise on pages 36–9, except this time keep your new understanding of intention in mind. Pause long enough – and with maximum curiosity and attention before you move – to try to detect your intention as it unfolds. Make your intention explicit, as in 'Now I will lift my arm', and then attend to how this unfolds.

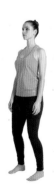
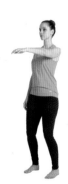
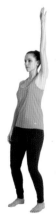
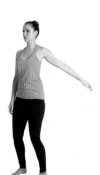

# Awareness of intention in others

In tai chi and other martial arts, gaining awareness of our own intentions is a way of attuning to the intentions of others.

Interestingly, the brain engages the same neural networks when *we* intend to move as those it uses when we observe *someone else* moving.[11] For example, if you see a friend reach for a glass of water, mirror neurons in your brain respond as if you were about to reach for the glass yourself. In your mind, you can have the experience of picking up the glass, too, but without the final motor execution. Your mind becomes a sort of 'simulator' for someone else's actions, enabling you to make a 'best guess' about the intentions of the other person.

So, in this example, you might well guess that your friend is thirsty.

This neural overlap develops at a young age. When we are infants, our own burgeoning ability to make intentional movements is the first rung on the ladder to understanding that other people have control over their actions, too. Once we realize this, we can start to be curious about what drives their behaviour (actions).[12] Our own movement helps us to understand the nature of other people; while the movement of other people helps us to understand ourselves

Have a go

## Notice your intention

Improving your awareness of changing posture is particularly valuable in improving your interactions with other people. As you become more aware of your intentions – and the sensations that arise in the seconds before you fulfil them – you also increase your sensitivity to the intentions of others. Focusing on our own posture changes and noticing how these influence or respond to those of other people deepens your powers of empathy. This is explored in more detail in Chapter 6.

For now, one good way to practise observing your intention to move is to stay mindful during changes in your posture. For example, as you intend to move from sitting to standing, or the other way round, or from lying to sitting, attend closely to the sensations that unfold in those nanoseconds before you begin the movement itself. Even if you don't want to change your posture, you could turn your attention to the intention to move your hand to turn the page of the book or to reach for a cup of tea.

## Stress and empathy

Our ability to mind-read (to understand, explain and predict the behaviour of others) is compromised during times of stress. Consider for a moment how in your own life your ability to communicate effectively breaks down when you feel under pressure. This is because you are too busy dealing with your own internal rumblings to tune in to the movements of other people. Stress tends to take us out of our bodies, into the thinking, doing space, which makes it hard for us to connect with others.

(through observing how others move in response to our own actions) and also others (we read and interpret others' movements in order to understand what they are thinking, feeling and intending).

### Intention and mind-reading

Overall, the developing infant is a highly tuned intentionality detector. At three months of age, infants can reliably detect the difference between things that move of their own will (with intention) and those that do not.[13]

This 'intention detector' is an early cognitive milestone necessary for the development of a sophisticated mind-reading system that comes

Tuning in to your intentions helps you

to understand how and why you act the

way you do.

online at about age four. Starting with the basic coding of intention via movement, we learn to make more abstract inferences about people's thoughts, beliefs and desires – intentions at the cognitive and emotional level.

We use this ability all the time as we negotiate the busy transport systems of our major cities, moving in large numbers without bumping into each other both on foot and in cars. Our brains are constantly reading the intentions of others in relation to how and where they are moving and adapting our actions to allow co-operative transit (just like in the Have a Go exercise, below).

BMT exercises help you to tap in to the several seconds of neural activity that occur before you actually move, which means that mindful movements can help you to experience your intentions fully. The more you practise tuning in to your intentions this way, the more familiar you can become with not only your detailed, specific intentions, but also with your intentions in a broader context, helping you to understand how and why you act the way you do.

## Walk in another man's shoes

As you walk down the street, turn your attention to the person in front of you. Mimic their body movement, posture and gait as closely as you can. Try to put yourself 'into' that person's body. Try the same thing with someone else of a different age. How does walking in someone else's shoes help you to connect with them, understand them or make inferences about their life, attitude and emotional state?

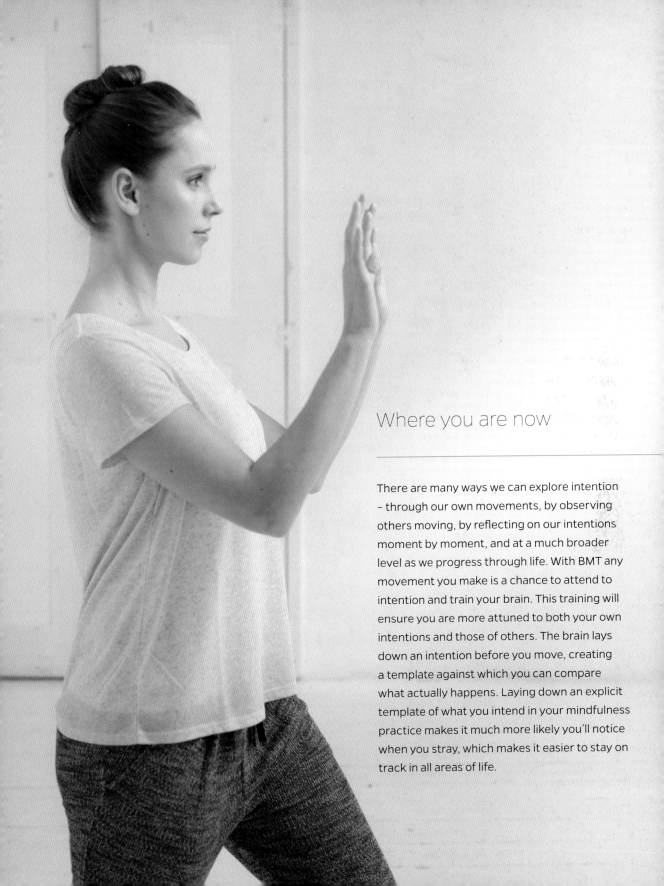

## Where you are now

There are many ways we can explore intention – through our own movements, by observing others moving, by reflecting on our intentions moment by moment, and at a much broader level as we progress through life. With BMT any movement you make is a chance to attend to intention and train your brain. This training will ensure you are more attuned to both your own intentions and those of others. The brain lays down an intention before you move, creating a template against which you can compare what actually happens. Laying down an explicit template of what you intend in your mindfulness practice makes it much more likely you'll notice when you stray, which makes it easier to stay on track in all areas of life.

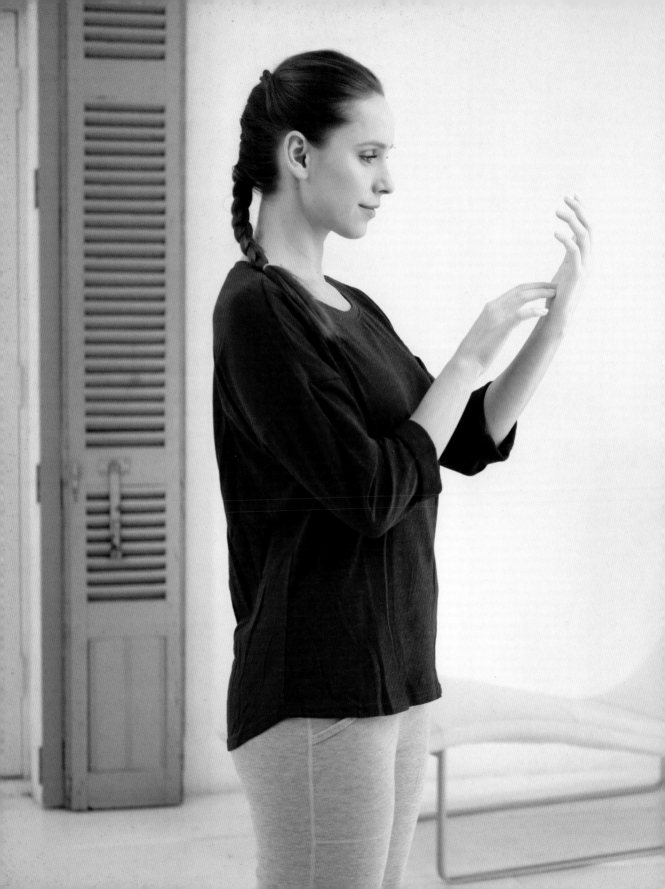

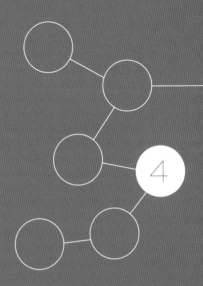

# Attention

In this chapter I'll explore the role of attention in mindfulness practice, using BMT exercises – and so the body – to help you to grasp key concepts. Deliberately training our attention through mindfulness of the body not only improves focus and clarity, it also helps us to regulate our emotional states, with huge benefits for our professional and personal lives.

The first step is to discover how we can train our brains by choosing where we place and move our attention. I'll show you how your focus can be narrow or wide, and under what conditions the lens of attention changes. We'll also explore how this training enables us to release the grip of emotions when we are stressed, and helps us to understand that we are more than just our pain, sadness or frustration.

# What is attention?

If we really want to engage with our experiences we need to stay with them, pay full attention to them and learn to notice when our attention wanders. This enables us to choose where we focus our attention, bringing some discipline to our naturally unruly minds.

I n Western psychology there are several different types of attention, shown in the diagram below.[1] These are alerting, orienting and executive attention. Each of these attention types has a dedicated neural network, which means we have three sets of 'attention muscles' to work on.

① **Alerting attention** refers to the system we engage when something – a sound somewhere nearby or a thought – catches our attention. It's the 'Hey, what's that?' signal that in times gone by would have brought into focus something relevant to our survival. This system means we are ready to be made aware of important information in the environment. If you were to hear a loud crash in another room while reading this book, your alerting system would be triggered. Even today, alerting attention is essential in certain situations (such as when you sense an oncoming danger on the road), but it can be distracting if you are, for example, focusing on incoming emails or Facebook 'pings' when you should be working or playing with your children!

Mindfulness training can teach you to detect when your mind moves in this very rapid way. While some of this movement is outside your control, much of it is habitual.

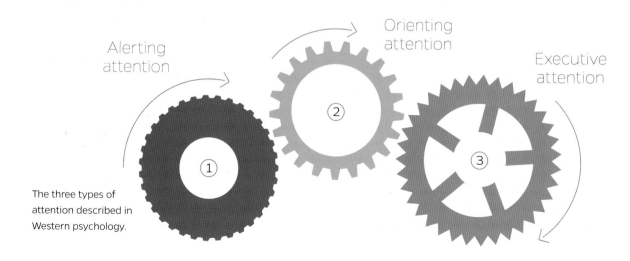

Alerting attention

Orienting attention

Executive attention

The three types of attention described in Western psychology.

## The ten stages of attention training

Although we have identified three types of attention, Buddhism describes many more, as a result of thousands of years of practice. In his excellent book *The Attention Revolution*,[2] author and contemplative scholar Alan Wallace details ten stages of attention development, ranging from directing attention to the breath (Stage 1) through to training in attentional stability and vividness to achieve a calm tranquillity of mind (Stage 10). Even reaching Stage 2 (maintaining full focus on an object for one minute without distraction) is beneficial, and someone who practises mindfulness regularly, but who lives in the 'real' world with a family, job and myriad other responsibilities, might only ever reach Stage 3 or 4. Going beyond Stage 4 requires a vocational commitment to attention training, including extended silent retreat practice – that is, training your attention in an environment with as few distractions as possible for months or even years.

② **Orienting attention** is used when we want to focus on one thing, to the exclusion of all others. Choosing to read these words requires you to orient your attention to the page, reducing the amount of attention you give to visual processing of the table, or the floor around you. This attentional system is much slower, and more effortful, but can easily be trained with mindfulness practice.

③ **Executive attention** is the most refined attention system, as it is the channel through which we take control voluntarily over our attention and experience. When executive attention kicks in, we have to let go of our focus on one thing in order to shift it to something else. This is what you practised when you disengaged from mind-wandering and refocused on bodily sensations. We use this kind of attention when we resolve conflicts between thoughts, feelings and actions; it enables us to reason. It brings objects into conscious awareness, so that we can manipulate them in a way that serves our goals and it helps us to inhibit (or reject) stimuli that no longer serve our purpose.

In your brain, the anterior cingulate cortex, a key region of the frontal lobe, is involved in executive attention. The connection of this region of the brain with other key frontal lobe regions changes even after a short training programme.[3] This region seems to work differently in those with meditation experience, responding more strongly compared with control participants in breathing meditation practice.[4] The cingulate cortex is also intimately connected with emotion-governing brain areas, which is why high emotion stops us from focusing.

'Arousal' refers to a state of wakefulness in the mind–body system. This is the 'how' rather than the 'what' part of attention. It is this type of attention we refer to when we ask ourselves during our mindfulness practice 'What is the quality of my attention? Is it dull? Sleepy? Relaxed? Agitated? Lax? Vivid?' We modulate this alertness deliberately when we begin mindfulness practice, putting the body into an 'alert but relaxed' state (pulling the spine upward, creating a sense of alertness, then releasing muscle tension).

# Training attention

In BMT we seek to discover what we can do right now – in the midst of our busy everyday lives – to train our attention, using the moving body as our main learning tool. The face, connected to a complex brain region, is particularly helpful as an area of focus.

The first step in learning how to train our attention is to understand how we can choose to move it around the body, learning as we do so more about what captures our attention. Eventually, it's possible to gain mastery over our attention system.

The following series of exercises will help you to start training your attention. By engaging with them, you will get to know your body at a much deeper level, as well as learn more about the signature of your mental movements – the times when you allow things other than the bodily sensations to capture your attention.

## Welcome to your face

If you have ever completed the traditional MBSR (Mindfulness Based Stress Reduction) or MBCT (Mindfulness Based Cognitive Therapy) programme you will be familiar with the body scan – a 45-minute exercise in which you systematically scan the body from the little toe to the head. The body scan targets all three types of attention (see pages 76–7), requiring you to orient attention to the body, sustain attention in the face of alerting distractors and monitor the whole endeavour to ensure you are on track.

BMT takes this practice further. In BMT the aim is not only to train the attention, but also to understand

---

**Have a go**

## Feel your brain in your hands

Using your hands as a focus enables you to sense how much larger the area of the brain for the hands is than, say, the part controlling the knee. Have a go now. Spend a few moments paying attention to your hands and notice the sensations in them. Then, spend a few moments paying attention to your knee. What did you discover?

You can also experiment with left and right sides. We are often strongly right- or left-handed, which means that there will be more brain dedicated to the dominant hand. See if you can detect this difference now by really paying attention as you switch your focus between the sensations in your left and right hands.

and employ the underlying neuroanatomy to help maximize your learning and optimize your practice. In addition, the more traditional body scan does not allow for spending time on the one area of your body where there is so often a wealth of sensations to feel – your face.

## The face and the brain

There are disproportionately large areas of your brain dedicated to both your face and your hands (see Have a go, opposite).The diagram below shows that huge swathes of the somatosensory cortex code facial information. This brain region is particularly large because our control over our facial muscles needs to be fine-tuned in order to allow us to speak, and also to communicate our emotions using our facial expressions. A constant flood of information flows between our face and this region of the brain, and this makes it an excellent subject for attention training.

In the exercise on pages 80–81 you'll move your attention around your face, learning to consciously orient it. Using your face rather than your whole body means you can practise the exercise anywhere, and you don't need to be lying down. Furthermore, working with a body part that is connected to such a large and complex brain region increases the training potential of the exercise.

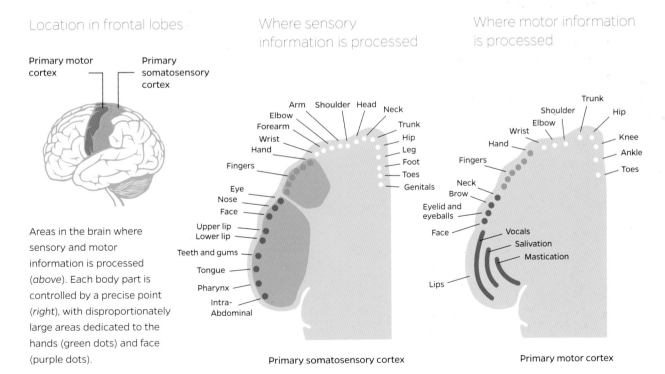

Location in frontal lobes

Where sensory information is processed

Where motor information is processed

Primary motor cortex
Primary somatosensory cortex

Areas in the brain where sensory and motor information is processed (*above*). Each body part is controlled by a precise point (*right*), with disproportionately large areas dedicated to the hands (green dots) and face (purple dots).

Arm  Shoulder  Head  Neck
Elbow
Forearm
Wrist
Hand
Fingers
Eye
Nose
Face
Upper lip
Lower lip
Teeth and gums
Tongue
Pharynx
Intra-Abdominal
Trunk
Hip
Leg
Foot
Toes
Genitals

Primary somatosensory cortex

Trunk
Shoulder  Hip
Elbow
Wrist
Hand
Fingers
Neck
Brow
Eyelid and eyeballs
Face
Lips
Knee
Ankle
Toes
Vocals
Salivation
Mastication

Primary motor cortex

# Let's practise:
# mindfulness of the face

This exercise, which should take 5 to 10 minutes, is intended as a formal practice, but actually you could practise it anywhere and at any time: try for five or six times a day (that adds up to 25–30 minutes of mindfulness a day!). You'll notice that each time you practise, your ability to maintain your focus increases and the exercise becomes easier. Whether you try it at work, on the bus, in the park or at home, slow down and before you begin set your intention as to whether you're using it as formal attention-training practice or informal 'checking in'.

① Sit in a comfortable position allowing your hands to rest on your lap to support the weight of your arms and shoulders. Ideally, close your eyes, but you can leave them open if closing them isn't safe (if you're driving, for example). Take three smooth and continuous breaths, setting your intention for your mind to be alert and your body relaxed.

② Deliberately focus your attention on your forehead. Scan this region with your 'mind's eye', either horizontally (between your hairline and your eyebrows) or vertically (across your forehead from left to right).

③ See if you can feel your eyebrows from the inside – can you determine where they start or stop? Are there more sensations toward the middle of your brows or more toward the outsides? If you can't feel any sensations at all, slowly raise your eyebrows up and down. Focus on the sensations in your eyebrows as you move them, then stop moving them and focus your attention on them. Keep your focus on your eyebrows, even if sensations are weak or absent.

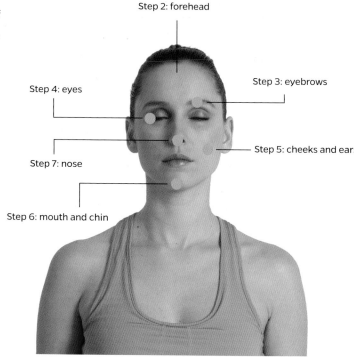

Step 2: forehead

Step 3: eyebrows

Step 4: eyes

Step 5: cheeks and ear

Step 7: nose

Step 6: mouth and chin

④ Now attend to your eyes and the region of your face around your eyes, including your eyelids, lashes and eyeballs, and the small muscles around the outsides of your eyes. Can you sense these muscles dropping or relaxing? Focusing your attention on your eyes themselves, do they feel dry or watery? Are they sore or tired? Try some mindful blinking.

⑤ Move your attention to your cheeks and ears. Can you detect sensations in the fleshy part of your cheek? Can you feel your cheek bones? What can you notice about the sensations on the insides and outsides of your cheeks – focus on one cheek and then the other, observing how you need to shift (orient) your attention to one side or the other. Release and relax the muscles that lie just below your ears, where your jaw begins, allowing your mouth to open slightly if this feels natural.

⑥ Deliberately move your attention to your mouth and chin. What can you notice that is hard or soft on the inside of your mouth, and then on the outside of your mouth? Can you notice where the inside portion of your lips becomes the outside portion?

Where is there moisture? Dryness? Can you detect any difference in the hard sensations of your teeth contrasted with the soft sensations from your tongue and lips?

⑦ Finally, move your attention to your nose, engaging with the sensations of your nostrils (can you feel the air against them as you breathe?), as well as those of the inside and outside parts of your nose. Finish the exercise by paying attention to three smooth continuous breaths, then open your eyes.

Be
curious

## Now try this ...

In this exercise you deliberately moved your attention around the face. Next time, try moving your attention from the bottom of your face to the top, or from the left to the right, or even from the front to the back (travelling from your face through your head and brain to the back of your head). The aim is to train your attention to go where *you* want it to go.

## Using your face to help you to let go

The illustration below shows the wealth of muscles that help you to form your facial expressions, and to move your mouth so that you can talk. In the previous exercise you may have started to get an idea of the sensations from these myriad facial muscles. In particular, around your eyes and the hinges of your jaw lie areas where you tend to hold tension and stress. It's here that you may have best been able to sense what happens when you 'let go'. But remember, in mindfulness, you are training to be okay with whatever is there, so it may just be you notice 'Wow, that's really tight.'

How you feel as you let go of the tension in these muscles is the same as the feeling of letting go you might aim to cultivate in your mind. This sense can be felt when you reduce the amount of constriction and struggle associated with your mental experiences.

Mindfulness aspires to an attentive state of mind – one that is alert but also relaxed. Too much alertness results in a type of strained or forced concentration, which could show up in your face as frowning and squinting. You'll probably find this kind of over-attention exhausting after a while.

If you notice that you're straining or tightening your face, try pausing and deliberately releasing your facial muscles, then check the quality of your

## Key muscles of the face

Becoming aware of the muscles that control your facial expressions will help you to pay attention to them and

relax the areas where you are holding stress. It will also increase your emotional awareness.

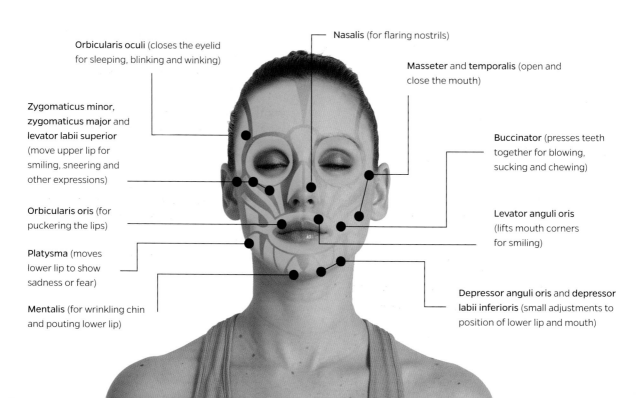

Orbicularis oculi (closes the eyelid for sleeping, blinking and winking)

Zygomaticus minor, zygomaticus major and levator labii superior (move upper lip for smiling, sneering and other expressions)

Orbicularis oris (for puckering the lips)

Platysma (moves lower lip to show sadness or fear)

Mentalis (for wrinkling chin and pouting lower lip)

Nasalis (for flaring nostrils)

Masseter and temporalis (open and close the mouth)

Buccinator (presses teeth together for blowing, sucking and chewing)

Levator anguli oris (lifts mouth corners for smiling)

Depressor anguli oris and depressor labii inferioris (small adjustments to position of lower lip and mouth)

attention and your mind. As you release your eye, cheek and jaw muscles around your face, you'll find that you also relax your tendency to grip on to your thoughts.

## Reading someone's mind

Have you ever seen an emotion 'flash' across someone's face? This is perceived when your brain codes the muscle configuration that indicates that person's emotional state. These micro-expressions are the ones we try to suppress when we want to hide our true feelings. However, mindfulness empowers you to catch them in someone else, even if they appear for only a fraction of a second, and this ability can be trained.[5]

A habit of 'checking in' with your face and staying alert to your facial expressions can develop your sensitivity to the emotions of other people, as well as your own. Research has shown that when we see another person smile or frown, we too generate a small smile or frown in return. This is called 'emotion contagion'[6] and it evolved as a way to help us live successfully in large social groups, where there was an advantage for those who could understand what others were feeling, and act accordingly.

You may have experienced this – think of people you know who are routinely smiling and happy. What effect do they have on your own mood? Pay attention to this next time you interact with someone who is either very happy or very low. See if you can, with mindfulness, start to notice when your face mimics theirs.

## Change your face, change your mood

Equally, honing your awareness of your own facial expressions helps you to keep a check on your own mood and develop emotional self-awareness (a key skill of emotional intelligence). Have you ever noticed how just smiling can make you instantly feel happier? Try holding a pen clenched between your teeth. See how it lifts up the sides of your mouth as if you were smiling and has an instantly lifting effect on your mood.

On the other hand, holding a pen between your lips to create a frown can induce a negative mood.[7] In psychology, these effects are referred to as the 'facial feedback hypothesis'.

Next time you try the mindfulness of the face exercise on pages 80–81, try ending it with a little smile on your face and see what happens. Observe how your body influences your mind – and your mind influences your body.

The practice

### The attention spotlight

You can think of your attention as a spotlight, with the following properties:

○ it can move voluntarily (we can choose where to focus our attention);

○ it can have a small, narrow focus or a wide focus (and it changes both automatically and voluntarily);

○ it is subject to unintentional change – for example, some things, such as stressful events or strong emotions that hijack our attention, automatically change the focus of the spotlight;

○ we can use it to bring items into the foreground of our attention, while there are still things occurring in the background.

# The attention spotlight

You've learned that you can deliberately move your attention around your face (and by extension to any part of your body), even when there are many internal and external distractions. Now it's time to learn how to widen and narrow your focus at will.

T hink about a spotlight on the actors on a stage – sometimes the light shines over large parts of the stage and many actors, and sometimes it hones in on just one spot and a single player. Playing with your visual attention is a good way to experiment with the notion of the attention spotlight (see the summary box on page 83). For example, right now narrow your attention so that you are fully focused on just one **w o r d** on this page. Now, widen your attention to take in the whole page, the book, then the environment you're in and what is going on around you.

## Attention and the martial arts

Practitioners of martial arts commonly employ a wider, softer focus of attention. This type of attention combines the alertness and the relaxation you need to be ready for action, avoiding the exhaustion that comes from being overly alert. It's a bit like increasing peripheral vision – you can take in more information, but with less detail.

You can also take this approach with your internal attention, broadening and expanding your focus using your mind's eye. If you practise doing this successfully, you'll also find it easier to notice when you're constricting your mental vision.

## Brain workout

Mindfulness attention training repeatedly narrows, widens, narrows, widens and so on the focus of your mind – just as you might do repeated lifts and lowers to strengthen your arms in the gym. Regular practice of the BMT exercise on page 86 helps to counteract any sense of mental or physical constriction, and also to maintain a broad but alert attention for longer periods of time.

In turn, this can help you to see that your experience is more than just your internal thoughts, feelings and emotions, and more than your pain, anger, judging and ruminating; and that the world is more than simply 'me' or 'I'.

## Exercising the lens of attention

The exercise on page 86 is very similar to the Mindfulness of the Face exercise on pages 80–81. However, this time you'll be finding out which part of your attention system helps you to narrow and widen your focus.

Alert but relaxed attention in mind and body: a monk practising the ancient art of tai chi at a temple on Mount Tai, one of China's sacred mountains.

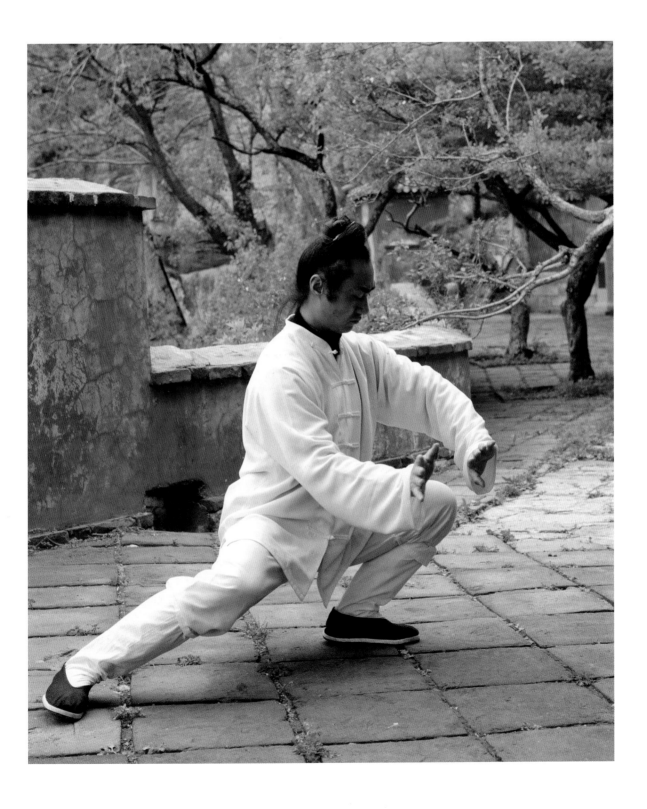

# Let's practise: changing the focus of the attention spotlight

Practise this exercise for 5 to 10 minutes in a quiet environment – it needs your complete focus.

① Settle into the exercise with a quick voluntary scan of your face from top to bottom, as you did in the exercise on page 80. Set your intention to be alert to the size of the lens of your attention, using the sensations of your face as the primary object of your attention.

② When you're ready, deliberately zoom your attention to the tip of your nose, becoming really curious about all the sensations you can feel there. Hold this attention for a few moments.

③ Deliberately choose to widen your attention from this point on your nose to the whole of your face. Note how you changed the lens of the spotlight, including observing what the widening motion feels like in your mind.

④ Now start to play: narrow your focus to the tip of your nose; widen it to your whole face; narrow it, widen it; narrow it, widen it. Keep practising back and forth, really working those attention muscles! Pay attention to your eyes. Our eyes and our attention system are so closely linked that when we work with internal attention, we often also move our eyes. The eye movement isn't necessary, so try to uncouple it from your internal attentional movement (this can take practice and succeeding is a sign of improved attentional control).

Be curious

## Now try this ...

The narrowing-widening exercise can be done with other parts of your body, of course. Try focusing on one finger or one toe, for example, and then expanding your attention again to encompass your whole hand or foot, and then your whole body.

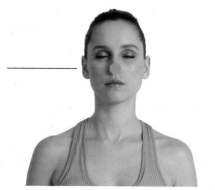

Attention on tip of nose —————

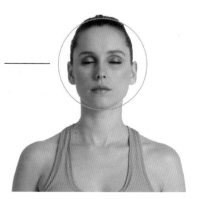

Attention widened to encompass whole face —————

# Importance of practice

The graceful and seemingly effortless movements of athletes or dancers are actually the result of hours of training and discipline. In order to achieve this level of effortlessness, all of us need to practise paying attention.

Mindfulness attention training is challenging, simply because most of us just aren't used to honing our brain activity in this way. Training the brain to be stronger in its focus is just like training any muscle in the body – at first, it will feel floppy and unco-ordinated, and it may even seem to 'protest' (it hurts, just like an out-of-condition muscle might) at such rigorous exercise and discipline. But, as with learning any new skill, when your efficiency increases, your pain and the effort needed will reduce. So persevere with the exercises – you will soon notice the difference! Routinely revisit your broader intentions with this practice to help keep you on track in a way that is meaningful for you.

## Practice makes perfect

A neuroimaging study of very experienced meditators[8] (with on average 44,000 hours of meditation practice) showed that their ability to pay attention was so well practised it had become effortless. Comparing very experienced monks to those with less training, the study asked monks to concentrate on a dot on a screen for an extended period of time. The study showed those in the early stages of training (the less experienced meditators) had more activation in the brain's attention network of their brains. The very experienced monks' attention network was in contrast relatively inactive. What once required much practice and effort had become effortless with training.

## Stroop task experiments

You may have heard of the 'Stroop effect', named after the researcher John Ridley Stroop. In Stroop task experiments, the name of a colour appears on a screen and it may or may not match the colour of the letters themselves. So, when the word 'red' appears, it might be written in blue ink. Or, it might be written in red ink. If the colour name and the lettering match, participants are asked to press a button. If they don't match, participants must hold back from pressing it.

A study I was involved in with colleagues from Brazil found that lay meditators were better able to pull back from making an incorrect cognitive judgment about non-matching words and colours, and inhibit their motor response for pressing the button, compared with control subjects.[9] To perform well on this task meditators used less of their frontal lobe than non-meditators. This suggests that their training had resulted in this area of the brain working more efficiently.

# Let's practise: holding the ball at shoulder height

In steps 1–12, you'll work to get the gist of the sequence. You'll be shifting your weight from your right to your left foot, and then from your left to your right foot, as you scoop your hand upward to shoulder height, as if you are holding a ball. If your weight is on your left foot, your right hand is holding the ball (and vice versa). Your body moves in a gentle fashion, left and right and slightly up and down.

Move on to step 13 to start to train your attention more precisely. You'll move a narrow attentional focus to your feet, waist and midsection, and then to your hands. Finally, shift your attention to your breath and then widen it to your whole body. Close your eyes if you feel comfortable, but if you're a beginner you might prefer to keep them open.

① Start in the tai chi standing posture, feet facing forward, knees slightly bent, pelvis tucked under slightly and with an alert but relaxed posture through your torso. Let your hands rest by your sides, palms down and fingers pointing forward.

② Begin by shifting your weight to your left foot. As you do so, rotate your right wrist so the palm turns inward, letting your palm push the air across the front of your body as your weight shifts. Throughout the movement to the left, keep your left hand near your left hip, palm facing the ground.

①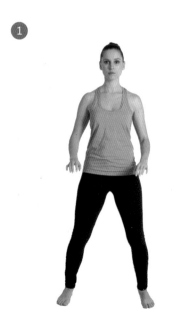

②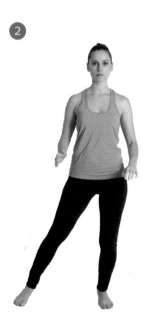

③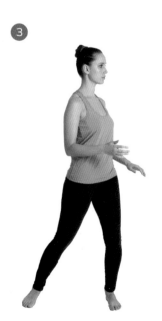

③ Once you have shifted your weight as far as you can, begin to turn your waist, 'dragging' your right hand even further until you reach the limit of the waist turn.

④ Now begin to peel up the right foot, until you are on the right tip toe creating a lifting movement (the right leg will extend, allowing the body to rise up). Keep rotating the wrist as you elevate the body, with the right hand eventually reaching shoulder height, palm facing upward to the sky, as if lifting and holding a ball. Pause and hold this position before you reverse the movement.

⑤ Rotate your right hand until the palm is facing downward, as you begin to connect the side of the right foot to the floor. As the foot reconnects you will naturally lower your hand. Work from the legs first and allow your hand to follow.

⑥ As your right foot reconnects to the floor, from the toe, to the ball of the foot to the whole foot down, shift your weight onto the right side and allow your right hand to rotate inward as your palm brushes the air across your body.

⑦ Regain the starting position. Now you will repeat the sequence of movements, shifting the weight to your right foot.

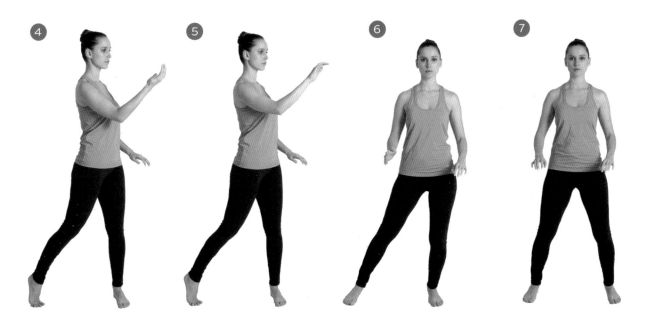

# holding the ball at shoulder height (continued)

8 As you shift your weight to your right foot, rotate your left wrist so the palm turns inward, letting your palm push the air across the front of your body as your weight shifts. Throughout the movement to the right, keep your right hand near your right hip, palm facing the ground.

9 Once you have shifted your weight as far as you can, begin to turn your waist, 'dragging' your left hand until you reach the limit of the waist turn.

10 Now begin to peel up the left foot, until you are on the left tip toe creating a lifting movement (the left leg will extend, allowing the body to rise up). Keep rotating the left wrist as you elevate the body, with the left hand eventually reaching shoulder height, palm facing upward to the sky, as if lifting

and holding a ball. Pause and hold this position before you reverse the movement.

11 Rotate your left hand until the palm is facing downward, as you begin to connect the side of the left foot to the floor. As the foot reconnects you will naturally lower your hand. Work from the legs first and allow your hand to follow.

12 As your left foot reconnects to the floor, from the toe, to the ball of the foot to the whole foot down, shift your weight onto the left side, allow your left hand to rotate inward as your palm brushes the air across your body.

13 Regain the starting position. As you continue moving through the sequence, attend to the

Repeat the sequence to the right

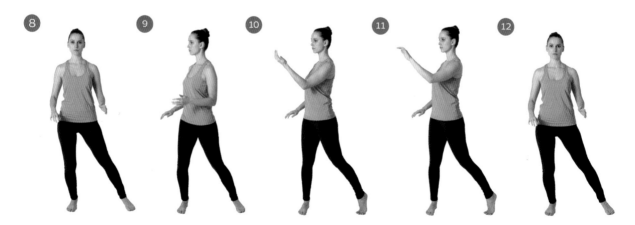

following aspects of the body in turn. Start by bringing a narrow focus of attention to your feet on the floor. Notice any change in pressure through your soles as you shift your weight. Attend to the timing of your weight shift and consequent changes in the sensations. Notice any difference between your left and right foot in terms of stability, balance, pressure and contact. As you shift to one side, become aware of how your other foot lifts up from the heel first, until you can feel your big toe touching the floor. As you reverse the movement, first feel your big toe on the floor, then the ball of your foot, then your heel. Notice how you can attend to these as three separate sensations unfolding over time (toe, ball, heel). When you change direction, observe the reversing of these actions – lifting the heel, peeling up the ball of the foot and touching the floor with your big toe.

(14) Now attend to your knee and pelvis as you continue moving. Shift your attention up one leg, noticing what the rest of the leg is doing. Focus on whether there is a slight bending and straightening of your knees. What is the most comfortable and useful point in the movement for this to occur? Experiment. As you shift your weight to one side, look for the 'shadow of the knee' over your toe – this tells you your knee and toe are aligned. Adjust your movement so that it is graceful and easy in whatever way works for you. As you shift your weight to the other leg, what sensations do you notice in your pelvis? Perhaps you notice the hardness of your bone and the way your pelvis moves as a single unit. Stay with these sensations, paying attention to the link between the weight shift and the movement of the pelvis. Try going more slowly.

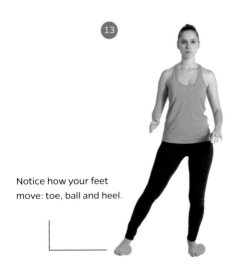

13

Notice how your feet move: toe, ball and heel.

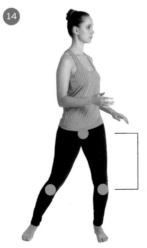

14

Be alert to your knees and pelvis.

# holding the ball at shoulder height (continued)

⑮ Shift your attention to your waist. This is the region above your hip bone and below your rib cage. See how you have to deliberately disengage from your pelvis to move your waist. Here, you can start to notice the way a turn in your waist follows your weight shift. If possible, separate the sensations of your hip and waist and experiment with how far you can turn your waist. Once your weight has shifted, stabilize through your leg and hip and allow your waist to turn freely from this position of stability. As you turn your waist, keep your arms relaxed and you'll notice you can execute much of your hand and arm movement through the waist movement itself. This is a really important aspect of tai chi practice – it's quite a lazy art that aims to do less and less to optimize movement. You'll notice you'll need to move your arm less if you can attend to the turn in your

waist and relax. Your waist will turn your torso and shoulders and your arm will follow naturally. As you turn your waist, be alert to the sensations in your rib cage, the muscles through your back, and the tactile sensations of your clothes. At the very end of the waist turn, allow your foot to come up onto your big toe. In essence your sequence is: weight shift, waist turn, and pushing off the floor with your big toe.

⑯ Now attend to your hands. As you push off the floor with your big toe, you might notice you're rising up slightly, straightening (but not locking) your knee. At the same time your hand will also start to lift up. As the waist turn allows the hand to travel from side to side, so this push off the floor allows the hand to be raised up slightly. You just need to get the hand in the right position to optimize what your body

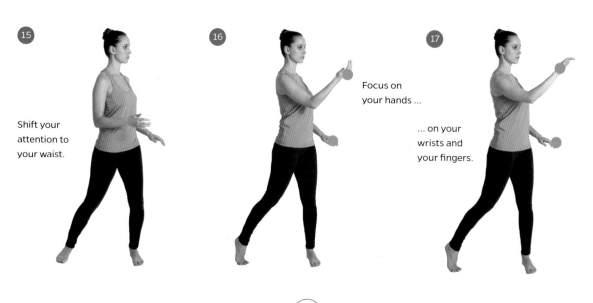

15

Shift your attention to your waist.

16

Focus on your hands ...

17

... on your wrists and your fingers.

is doing. Your palm should face up on the way up; down on the way down. Starting with your hand palm downward and positioned by your hip, turn it inward, as if scooping. Stay relaxed, allowing your shift in weight and turn in your waist to do the work. How far can your hand move without you actually moving it? As you push off the floor with your toe, turn your palm upward, as if you are now holding a ball in your palm. Use just enough power to lift your hand to shoulder height. Watch out for striving and trying to do too much. If you see this, don't worry – just notice this tendency and see if you can pull back, activating those motor inhibition networks in your brain.

(17) As you begin to reverse the movement, turn your palm over to face the floor. Take your attention into all those bones that make up your wrist and really feel the turning movement, staying curious about how and what initiates the movement. Keep your fingers as relaxed as possible to allow you to experience directly the mechanics inside your wrist and forearm. Really feel the articulation of the wrist joint as you turn the hand over. Take your attention to each finger individually and explore any sensations from your palm to the tip of each finger. As the ball and then heel of your foot reconnect to the ground, turn over your hand and allow it to travel down back to your waist. As your weight shifts to the other side, your other hand will start to lift up and hold the ball. If your mind wanders, just bring it back over and over again. Remember you might need to reset your intention (perhaps saying gently to yourself 'hand, hand').

(18) Shift your attention to your breath, keeping your movement as smooth and graceful as possible. Bring your attention to your in-breath (through your nose) and your out-breath (through your mouth). There is no need to change your breathing rate, but see what happens if you breathe in as you lift your hand up, and breath out as your hand comes down. Go at a pace that is comfortable for you, where you can be relaxed and graceful without any striving. Bring your attention to the sensation of your breath entering and exiting your body, in the region of your nose and mouth. Bring attention to the movement of your breath in your body, and the expansion and contraction of your rib cage. Notice the transition between in- and out-breath and how that is linked to your hand movement.

(19) Now widen your attention to your whole body and your breath. See how you have to widen the lens of attention to include many more objects. Your focus is less precise in this scenario, but can take in more information. Continue with this wide focus for about 6–10 more movements. Be alert to mind-wandering and refocus your attention to your body.

(20) To end the exercise, with full attention and intention, cease your movement. Come back to your starting position and stand for a few moments, noticing the contrast in your body between movement and stillness. Your movement may continue to occur even when your body is still, so don't rush to finish. Just pause. What is different in your body and mind having done this exercise?

# Attention and emotion disruption

Attention training equips you to take appropriate action when high emotions or stressful situations threaten to overwhelm you.

Our brains are capable of all sorts of amazing things – planning, analysing, monitoring and manipulating information. Many of these so-called 'executive functions' are managed by the frontal lobes. When we are calm and relaxed we can use the frontal lobes to their full extent. Our emotions arise from activation in the limbic system. When we are stressed or emotional, we use this primitive part of our brain. When the limbic system is activated the brain operates in a mode of freeze, fight or flight. The result is that our sophisticated thinking and strategic abilities are compromised as brain resources are occupied managing emotions. We engage fully with trying to control our emotional state, instead of focusing on the present.

## The brain under stress
Can you remember a time when you were really stressed or upset? What happened to your ability to communicate or think clearly? Did you become

## Effect of emotional disturbance

These illustrations show the brain during calm (*below left*) and stressful conditions (*below right*).

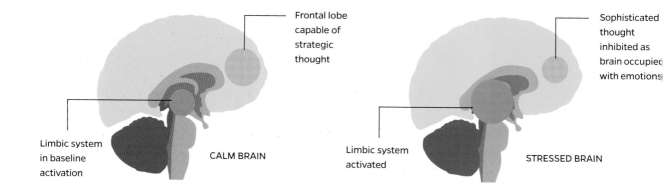

Frontal lobe capable of strategic thought

Limbic system in baseline activation

CALM BRAIN

Sophisticated thought inhibited as brain occupied with emotions

Limbic system activated

STRESSED BRAIN

snappy or did you garble your words? Stress inhibits the ability of the brain's frontal lobe to monitor speech. The limbic emotional system takes over and the frontal lobe goes offline – the brain can't waste energy thinking about others or planning how to be eloquent when there is danger or an urgent need to flee!

However, regular mindfulness training can boost the efficiency of the frontal lobes so that, even in the face of a strong emotion, you are better able to function in a considered way. Mindfulness gives you the ability to pause and to choose when you focus your attention, and how to respond, rather than react without thinking.

It is really important to understand that mindfulness training does not diminish or suppress emotion. In fact, it does the opposite – it encourages you to welcome your emotions and face them with simplicity and honesty, reducing emotional intensity and so disarming much of the additional suffering and anxiety that you yourself create around it.

## Effect of mindfulness on the brain

After mindfulness training, we can think strategically even when experiencing stress or high emotion.

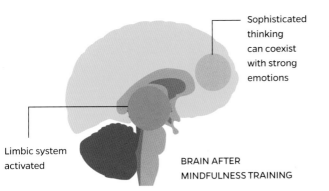

Sophisticated thinking can coexist with strong emotions

Limbic system activated

BRAIN AFTER
MINDFULNESS TRAINING

Mindfulness encourages you to welcome your emotions and face them with simplicity and honesty, reducing emotional intensity.

## High emotion and mindfulness

Working with mindfulness gives you several options as to where in the body you direct your attention when you are faced with strong emotions. In the early stages of mindfulness training it's helpful to use mindfulness of the moving body as the training tool (as we primarily do in this book), because the sensations of your moving body capture and hold your attention more easily – keeping you in the present moment. With a little more training and confidence, however, you will be able to bring your attention directly to how the emotion manifests in sensations in your body. When you can do this, you're ready to stop labelling your emotional experiences as 'pleasant' or 'unpleasant' and instead cultivate a genuine, present moment acceptance of all aspects of your emotions. Can you treat happiness and sadness just the same? This doesn't mean that you don't feel these emotions, it just means that you don't get drawn into them, overwhelmed by them and compromised by them.

## When the going gets tough, hit your feet

The sensations you experience in the soles of your feet can really hold your attention. The exercise on pages 96–7 is a certain way to connect to your body even in times of genuine emotional upheaval – practise and it will help you the next time you start to feel annoyed or even angry, allowing you to literally 'stand' your feelings.

# Let's practise: mindfulness of the soles of the feet

Try this exercise with your shoes on or off, on different surfaces – sand and grass are ideal, but it's also good to do under your desk at work! Close your eyes for greater sensitivity to body sensations, but keep them open if you feel unstable or dizzy. If your eyes are open, keep your gaze still and broadly unfocused on an area just in front of you.

① Begin by positioning yourself in the tai chi standing posture, with your feet facing forward, knees slightly bent, pelvis tucked under slightly, arms relaxed and an alert but relaxed posture through your torso (see page 36).

② Take three smooth and continuous breaths and with each out-breath deliberately move your attention to the soles of your feet. You might get a sense of your mind 'dropping' down into your body all the way to your feet. Narrow your focus of attention and explore the soles of your feet,

focusing on the points of pressure and places where you can feel your body's weight through your feet. Explore the ball, heel, sides and top of your feet – either one at a time or both at the same time (try both ways). Notice how you are standing right now, without making any adjustments. What can you observe?

③ Slowly move your weight forward and backward onto the balls of your feet, then onto your heels. Do this with as little actual movement in your body as possible. Imagine that an onlooker would barely know you are moving, but *you* can feel the difference in the sensations from your body and your feet. Pay close attention to any changes in the sensations through your feet as you shift your weight forward and backward. Stay alert to how the sensations unfold over time. Checking in with the body, see what adjustments you can make to find more comfort or ease in your posture.

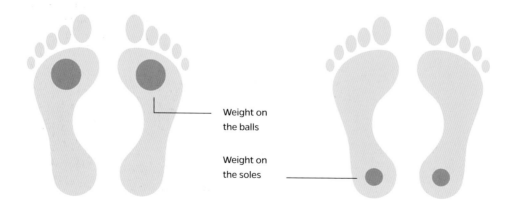

Weight on the balls

Weight on the soles

Be
curious

## Now try this ...

A variation on the exercise is to play with the timing of your weight distribution as you walk or run. As you step forward, take a micro-second to become aware of your foot hovering above the ground, just before you lower your weight into it and touch the floor. Be curious about the way you have executed the motor command to place your foot down, and consciously inhibited the instruction. By practising this you improve your ability to inhibit action at the cognitive and emotional levels. Notice also how you can break down your leg and feet movements even further. As you are walking or running, try to be aware of how movement and control through the front of the hip impact on the placement of the foot on the ground.

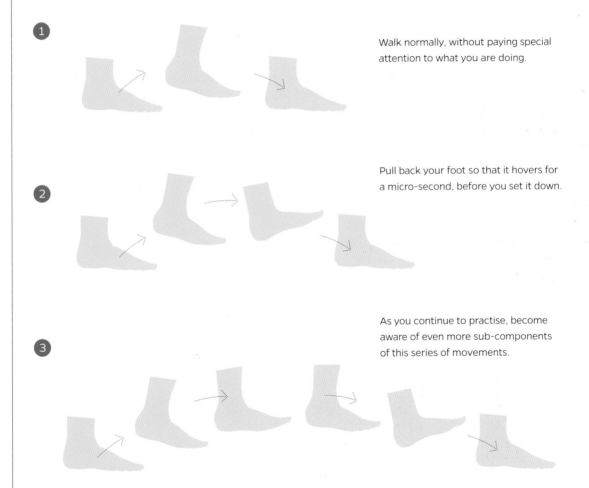

① Walk normally, without paying special attention to what you are doing.

② Pull back your foot so that it hovers for a micro-second, before you set it down.

③ As you continue to practise, become aware of even more sub-components of this series of movements.

## Overcoming stress

When you focus your mind on the movement of and pressure in your feet, several things happen. First, you voluntarily shift your attention to the incoming raw sensations in your feet, taking back control of your mind so that your emotions are no longer hijacking your attention.

Second, you attend to your bodily sensations, which keeps you in the present moment. Finally, as a result of both those things, you interrupt the unhelpful patterns of thinking that emerge when strong, negative emotions surge through you.

Your mindfulness practice also encourages you to recognize and accept that you have negative or unwanted sensations – including mental habits and raw emotions – and to move over and beyond them, so that your mindful focus is on something else. In this case, the something else is your feet, which are available to you at all times in your daily life – either for formal practice, or simply when you are running for a train or walking to the water cooler. Practising a little bit each day means you will have the confidence with these techniques when you are under pressure and really need them.

Have a go

## Make an empty step

In tai chi, shifting your weight from the left to the right foot means you are making one foot 'empty' and the other 'full'. An empty step is one in which your foot appears to be stepping, but you have not fully deployed your weight – perhaps because you've left 60, 70, 80, 90 or even 100 per cent of your weight with your other foot. How much weight you deploy is less important than knowing and being sensitive to the ratios in left and right.

Try this standing still in the queue at the supermarket or while waiting for the bus. Keeping both your feet on the ground, experiment with putting your full weight into one foot and then into the other. Stay acutely aware of how the weight shifts – where and when. Then, change the ratios (as often as you like).

Tai chi teaches that there are nine full points and one empty point of contact on the foot. Try the exercise on page 96 when you have your shoes off, or do it wearing martial arts soft shoes, to see if you can detect the nine points of contact as your feet meet the ground.

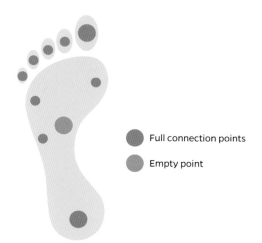

● Full connection points
● Empty point

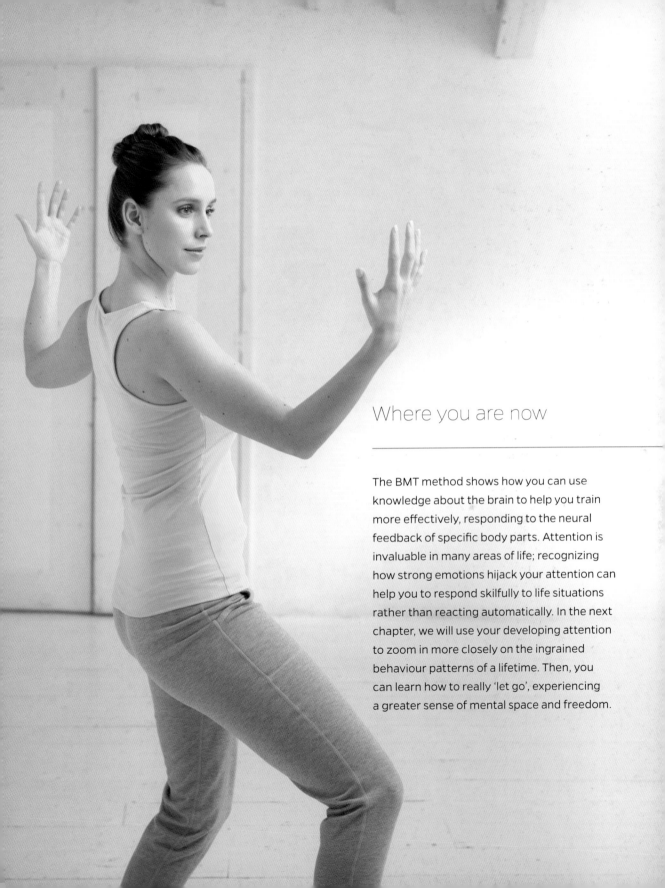

## Where you are now

The BMT method shows how you can use knowledge about the brain to help you train more effectively, responding to the neural feedback of specific body parts. Attention is invaluable in many areas of life; recognizing how strong emotions hijack your attention can help you to respond skilfully to life situations rather than reacting automatically. In the next chapter, we will use your developing attention to zoom in more closely on the ingrained behaviour patterns of a lifetime. Then, you can learn how to really 'let go', experiencing a greater sense of mental space and freedom.

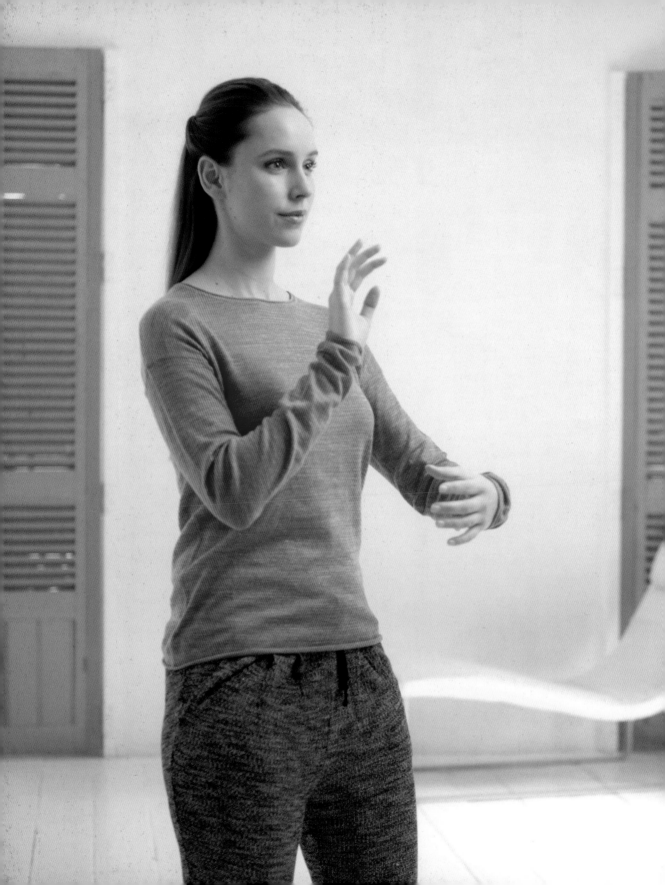

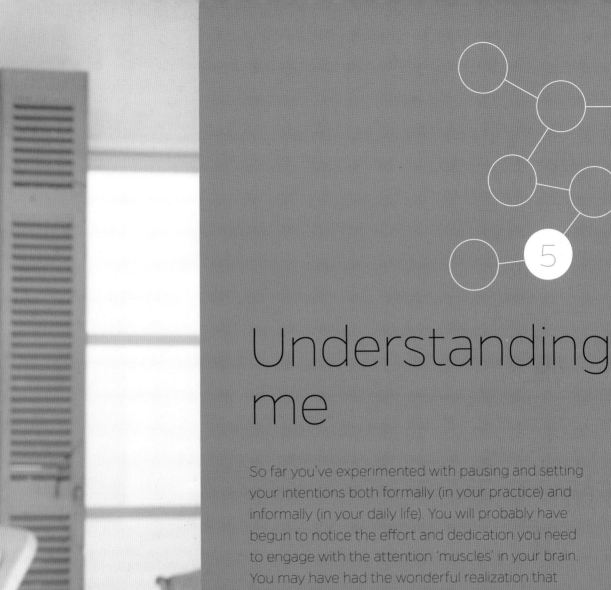

# Understanding me

So far you've experimented with pausing and setting your intentions both formally (in your practice) and informally (in your daily life). You will probably have begun to notice the effort and dedication you need to engage with the attention 'muscles' in your brain. You may have had the wonderful realization that through your hard work, your attention is wandering less. You may also have become more aware of painful reactions, and noticed the tendency to turn away from these as quickly as possible. This makes sense in the short term, but may be harmful in the longer term. In this chapter we're going to delve a little deeper into the mental processes that may seem like they are helping us, but have actually become energy sapping. You'll realize that avoiding negative experiences in fact prevents you from living life to the full.

# Wandering mind

The mind wanders in relatively predictable ways during mindfulness practice and throughout daily life, anticipating the future and reflecting on the past. Mundane ruminating is much easier to deal with than our deeply engrained mental responses.

A s you practised the exercises, you may have noticed your mind's tendency to move forward and backward in time. This might be thinking about something you will do later today or going back to the past, mulling over something that has happened. If you are noticing these mind states, you are doing brilliantly – you are catching your thoughts as they happen. However, now it's time to go deeper and work harder to manage your wandering mind.

Once you get into the habit of spotting when you have left the present, you will find that some types of mind-wandering are relatively easy to manage. Other times, however, you might observe very fast mind-wandering that takes you very far in your chain of thinking. This may represent more deep-seated mental habits that will require more investigation and patience. Mind-wandering is a natural function of the brain[1] but it can sometimes be highly automatic and unhelpful.[2] This is where mindfulness training really can help. Some mental habits may have been with you since your childhood years, representing old ways of trying to cope with emotional situations that are just not useful any more. If this is the case, you will need to investigate them closely and with kindness.

Experiencing your challenging mental states fully in your mind–body allows you to get to know their characteristics thoroughly. You'll learn when they like to emerge, and become highly curious as to where they sit in the temporal sequence of your mental patterns. You can ask yourself, 'What happens just before this habit gets triggered? And then what comes after that?' In Chapter 2 you watched your bodily sensations unfold over time; now you're going to do this with your thoughts, feelings and memories. Previously, you let go of attaching verbal labels and images to your thoughts and feelings, but the first step in this process is to quickly label your sensations (mental or physical) – try the exercise opposite.

## Mindfulness of sound

Close your eyes and set your intention to pay close attention to sounds anywhere in your environment. Observe how different sounds draw your attention to the left, the right, in front and behind. Pay attention to *how* your mind moves – how fast it flits from one sound to another, how it moves through space and how sounds trigger labels, images and trains of thought. Really investigate without trying to control the experience.

Have a go

# Let's practise:
# labelling mental sensations

In this exercise you will use your breath as the focus of your attention. When you label sensations, do so quickly – make your labels sharp and reliable. Practise for 5 minutes.

① Sit comfortably and quietly and take three breaths. Set your intention to pay attention to the mental and physical sensations that enter your awareness moment by moment with each of your three breaths. When you notice a sensation in your mind (for example, a thought, a memory, or an image) give it a very quick verbal label. For example, you might give the label 'sound' when you hear a sound, or 'future thought' when you notice you have started thinking about the emails you will send after practising this exercise. Immediately after you have given the label, come back to your breath.

② What did you notice? How easy or difficult was it to quickly label the phenomena and then come back to your breath? Notice how you can label in a broad way (for example, 'thought' or 'body sensation') or with more detail (for example, 'itching' or 'tingling' or 'future planning'). Did you get stuck trying to find a label? That's okay – just be aware of it for now, accept that there will have been sensations you missed while you were stumbling over this one, and know that labelling gets easier with practice.

Be curious

## Now try this ...

As a variation you could try using your body, or part of your body, as the anchor. Alternatively, you could work with no anchor – keeping your attention, moment by moment, focused on your mental phenomena (thoughts, memories, images). In either variation, as sensations arise, give them a quick label before dropping and seeing what next ... what next ...

Labelling sensations in mind and body as they unfold over time

You can label your experiences using general terms.

'Body sensation' → 'Thought' → 'Sound' →

You can also label your experiences using more specific terms.

Itch → Planning → Remembering →

## The bird watcher

My dearest friend can identify a bird from the slightest twitch. The process she went through to become an expert in bird watching is similar to what we aspire to in our mindfulness training. In the early stages, she would spot a bird, then hunch over a bird guide, checking the wings, the beak, the body shape and flight pattern to identify what it was. She engaged her full attention and curiosity as she checked each and every bird she saw – this was the learning process. As her expertise developed, she became able to identify the bird from its flight pattern alone and no longer relied on an overt label.

Just as my friend eventually learned to identify her birds by movement alone, so it is with detecting our mental habits. At first the movements in your mind are outside your awareness. The process of identifying and verbally labelling them helps you to bring these patterns to your conscious awareness, to discriminate between them and to know them better. Once you have developed this recognition skill, you can drop the overt labelling and detect habits based on the movement in your mind alone. Your speed at detecting these mental movements will increase the more you practise.

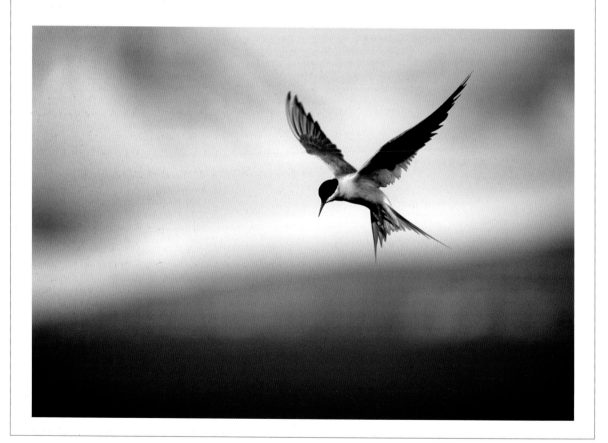

# Focus on the self

Now you have the tools to start studying your own mind. The more information about yourself you gather, the better able you will be to catch habitual reactions at an early stage and instead choose a new, lighter and less emotional response.

M indfulness for me is like a scientific training. To investigate ourselves thoroughly, we need to adopt the qualities of a good scientist – someone whose approach to discovery involves being observant, persistent and honest (a good detective or journalist are also examples). So, what qualities do we want to develop in order to understand ourselves?

**Curiosity** – because this motivates us to find out more

**Deep observation** – because we must be prepared to look again and again

**Honesty** – because learning involves a true reflection of ourselves

**Non-judgment** – because to be honest we have to accept what we see, not what we perceive or imagine or wish to be true

**Trust** – because we have to believe in the method and training process

**A beginner's mind** – because we can't shake judgment unless we approach ourselves with fresh eyes

**Open-mindedness** – because we might not like what we discover, but we must accept it just the same

When you can see what your mind is doing, thinking, imagining, you give yourself the choice to respond in new ways.

This process has already given you several tools – the ability to pause, explore your intention and focus your attention – that enable you to gather data about yourself. By repeatedly sampling your mental and physical sensations under different conditions and over time, you develop the capacity to observe what is *really* going on in your mind. When you can see what your mind is doing, thinking, imagining, you give yourself the choice to respond in new ways rather than repeating the same old patterns. This is where real freedom begins – particularly freedom from strong emotions.

## Catching emotions

Mindfulness gives us an opportunity to engage with the moments when our emotions threaten to overwhelm us, because it enables us to find out what is happening in the mind–body system just before the emotion is triggered, or just after. Your mindful exploration into your own sensations teaches you to greet your emotional responses by name and to label them – 'Ah, there is anger, tightening, constriction.' Verbally labelling our emotional experience is a way of putting on the brain's 'brakes', activating the right ventrolateral prefrontal cortex (see page 46), helping us to regulate our emotional experience.[3] Neuroscience research shows that putting feelings into words reduces the response of the emotional limbic system and recruits a circuit in the frontal lobe of the brain.[4] This includes the right ventrolateral prefrontal cortex, the region engaged when we overtly label an emotion. It works together with the medial prefrontal cortex, helping us to tone down our emotional reactions. Put simply, we use the frontal lobe to take charge of our emotions. Doing this mindfully requires us to be kind toward the emotion, give it some room to be seen and heard, but not let it take over. This is responding rather than reacting.

## Freeing up brain energy

Imagine being in the middle of a stampeding herd of wildebeest. Noise, hooves, sweat, dirt, fear – you are right in the thick of it, but desperately want to escape. You may try to take control of the situation – fighting and forcing your way to the edge of the herd to bring it under control. This strategy is possible but likely to be exhausting, and not sustainable.

Through teaching you to pull back, to release the urge to fight and control, mindfulness training shows you how to let go. You learn that you have the option to yield rather than push against the stampede. When you let go of the struggle, you not

Reflect on this

### What is stopping you?

Repeatedly asking yourself the question 'What stops me from being mindful?' can illuminate what triggers your mental habits and when. You might first explore external factors, the obvious being time or place. Where are you? At home or work? Is there a certain time of day that sets your mind wandering? Then, examine internal factors, such as feelings of boredom or fear.

My frequent answer when I ask myself this question is 'teaching other people to be mindful'. For many reasons, I find that the more I teach, the less I practise myself. When I realize this, I know it's time for me to revisit my intentions for my own practice. Remember that the moments when you are convinced you don't have time for mindfulness are exactly the times you need to pause and get into your body. Your body is with you all the time – so there is really no excuse.

only reduce your own stress and frustration, you also conserve valuable brain energy. This is a key principle in tai chi: yielding conserves energy and makes you more effective.

With practice, mindfulness enables you to identify the mental sequence of events that pulls you into the stampede in the first place. At first, you might not always be able to avoid the stampede, but over time you'll get better at recognizing repeated patterns of behaviour, and you'll catch yourself, saying 'Oh, am I doing that again?' As you increasingly engage with the habits you want to change, you can stop avoiding them and struggling against them.

# Mindful movement and mental habits

The way we move physically has much to teach us about our mental patterns; in particular, about how we cope with frustration.

earning new sequences in tai chi is a great way to find out more about our mental habits. This is because, faced with the challenge of completing a new sequence and perhaps not doing it perfectly the first time (or first few times), we might feel frustration, irritation or jealousy (what did you feel when you did the exercise on pages 88–93?). These reactions teach us about how we deal with adversity in general. However, frustration, in particular, is a natural part of the learning experience. In mindfulness it's what you do with this frustration that counts. Do you hang on to it? Or, do you let it go? Can you learn more about it? What does it feel like in your body? Where else does this emotion crop up in your life?

As you train your body, you'll get a clearer picture of your psychological profile. In my martial arts classes, my instruction to my students is, first, to clearly acknowledge that frustration is there, then to label and explore it quickly, then to release it (drop it), and finally to refocus intention and attention on the body. If possible, greet any particularly unpleasant feelings within you with a big hug, then in the next second refocus your attention on the task. If you bring the frustration from the last thing you were doing with you, you can't properly engage with the present task – so your frustration can only mount. The exercise on pages 108–109 allows you to focus on this.

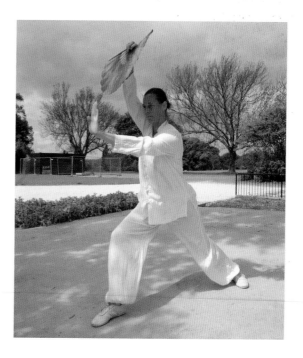

Learning new sequences is a journey that includes frustration, irritation, pride and joy – all these reactions help us to learn more about ourselves.

# Let's practise:
# cup of tea and paintbrush

I have taught this exercise in many settings, from corporate offices to psychiatric emergency rooms. It requires both the left and right hemispheres of your brain to be doing different things at the same time, so I've found that it frequently generates frustration! Practise it mindfully, in order to see where that frustration arises in body and mind, for 5 to 10 minutes at a time. Remember that throughout you need to go slowly (and then 50 per cent more slowly!) and observe how the mental and physical movement unfolds over time. Be alert to your intention to move, especially around transition points, and concentrate on where your attention

lies (and how it is distracted along the way). The exercise suggests a standing position, but you could practise it sitting, right now, if you like.

(1) Begin in the tai chi standing posture (see page 36). Relax your hips and lower back and allow your shoulders to sink. Take three smooth and continuous breaths to begin, and with each out-breath set your intention and bring your attention into the body.

(2) Raise your right hand to shoulder height. Remain aware of your intention travelling from your brain to your arm and initiate a movement of your left arm

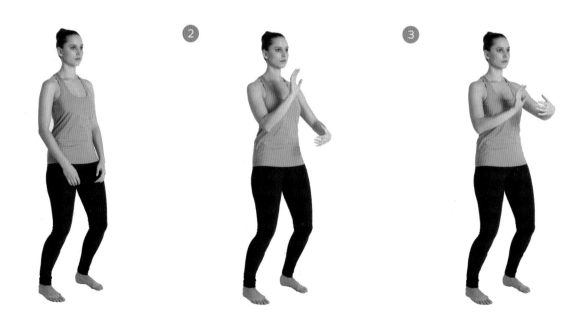

upward, with your hand in a grasping position – as if you were picking up a takeaway coffee cup. This is your 'cup' hand. At the same time, move your right hand downward, with your palm facing forward, keeping this hand closest to your body. This is your 'paintbrush' hand.

③ Your hands should pass by each other, palms facing, at the level of the middle of your chest.

④ Continue until your 'cup' hand reaches chin height and your 'paintbrush' hand reaches your belly button.

⑤ Now your 'cup' hand becomes the 'paintbush' hand and starts to travel downward, and the 'paintbrush' hand becomes the 'cup' hand and starts to travel upward. Always keep your 'paintbrush' hand closest to your body.

⑥ Continue with this sequence of movements. Notice what happens in the mind as you try something new – how did your mind react to the challenge of learning this movement? Is this a reaction you see elsewhere in your life at all? If you felt frustrated, at what point did this kick in? Observe how you narrowed and widened your attention to the physical movement and also how attentional focus was engaged by emotional or mental movements.

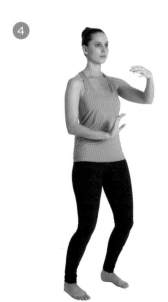

④

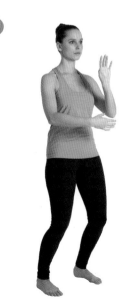

⑤

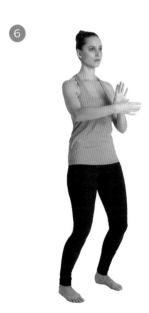

⑥

# Meeting and greeting mental monkeys

'Mental monkeys' are the unruly states of mind that distract our attention, reduce our potential and generally hinder our progress.

In martial arts training we use body work to access our 'mental monkeys'. These distracting and inhibiting mind states frequently come out when we are learning new routines, or when we are tired, fed up, angry and frustrated (usually with ourselves). Yet, like all things in martial arts practice, these monkeys are actually to be celebrated. Understanding and managing their characteristics is the key to reaching our full potential in life.

Monkeys are full of energy and curiosity, but not always skilful; sometimes they can even be vicious and cruel. Can we accept these characteristics without judgment? We can't blame a monkey for being cheeky – that is their nature. We can't get angry with monkeys even when they behave 'badly' – that's just how they are.

Whenever I notice I am getting caught up in judging my experience, I visualize a certain photograph of a monkey's face. (You might find an image of a monkey you can use as a screensaver to remind you of your mental monkey habits.) The photograph reminds me that our minds are like cheeky monkeys and that I shouldn't be too hard on myself. It also brings a smile to my face – and humour is vital for mindfulness practice (after all, the mind is a pretty crazy place and

it helps to have a lightness as we engage with it). During mindfulness, we aren't trying to stop or even change the monkeys, we are learning to engage with them.

## Which monkeys live with you?

In BMT we get to know our monkeys really well. They all have their own characters, but wear slightly different jackets. We learn not only their mental signatures, but also how they feel in our bodies.[5] I love author Martine Batchelor's description of these different monkeys,[6] and have added a few more of my own. You can often spot them by recognizing their favourite phrases: 'If only ...', 'Why?', 'What if?'

**Daydreaming monkey** gets lost in fantasyland. This monkey creates some lovely places for the mind to reside, making it particularly seductive as monkeys go, but its world is not reality.

**Rehearsal monkey** goes over and over what we will say, what they will say, then what we will say back ... This monkey often appears when someone has said or done something that has upset us. Rather than deal with unpleasant feelings, this monkey works out the sniping or witty retorts.

**Fabrications monkey** loves to make up stories that we end up believing. It's the monkey that says 'If only ...' Fabrications will probably end up believing its own stories, too.

**Judging monkey** is out of control! All over the place and super-critical, it judges everyone and everything ... usually negatively. Judging monkey appears so quickly we can't always detect it. It does not discern (which is reasoned form of judgment), but jumps to hasty and inaccurate conclusions and leaves us feeling tired and empty.

**Comparing monkey** likes to check how we are doing compared to everyone else and compared to how we were before, or want to be in the future. Consumer culture particularly exploits this monkey. When it comes to our emotions, it can really get us into trouble – emotions are ours and ours alone, and are manifested in the experience of that moment, so cannot be compared with the past or projected into the future, or compared with those of others.

**Planning monkey** loves to organize everything down to the last detail. It comes out when we try to sneak in a few 'to-do' lists while we are practising or paying attention to our breath. Planning monkey goes into overdrive when we are anxious, trying to simulate and plan responses for all different scenarios in order to regain a sense of control. However, its efforts are futile and we just end up exhausted, because even after all that planning there's still no certainty.

**Measuring and counting monkeys** are the 'bean-counting' monkeys of our mind. They check our

## Celebrate your mental monkeys

In martial arts there is a saying that the students who have the most balanced ying and yang are likely to be problematic. They have a natural talent and sail through the physical demands of the class, learning the techniques easily. These students do not receive the 'gift' of difficult practice and do not get to overcome so many psychological barriers (mental monkeys) during training. So, celebrate your monkeys – they are your greatest teachers!

progress against internal markers, to see if we are 'there' yet, but seeing as there is no 'there', these monkeys are just a huge waste of mental energy.

**'Should' monkey** tells us what we 'should' do, say, want ... Stay *very* alert whenever a should monkey appears – there's no such thing as 'should' and often should monkey has only criticisms to give.

**Analytical monkey** loves to puzzle things out. Keep a tight rein on this monkey, especially if you are an academic or a therapist or have been trained in any other analytical way, because this one gets endlessly caught up in working out *why* ...

When working with your mental monkeys, you will need patience, kindness, firmness, discipline and persistence – but most of all humour. Your mindfulness training will engage your attention and using the techniques you've learned so far, you can try to keep those naughty monkeys firmly in check.

## Cross your arms

Right now, cross your arms. Now cross them the 'other way'. What did you notice? When we start to change habits, even simple physical ones, we realize that we have to apply effort and fully engage our attention to do so. When it comes to mental monkeys, it is often much easier to keep doing the same thing, allowing the same monkeys to have their way. We can quieten them only by dedicating our attention to the task.

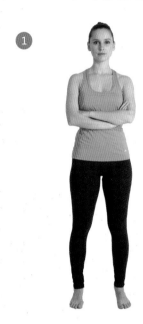

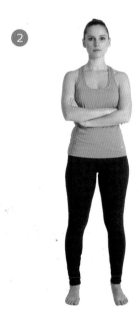

## Creating new habits

Much like the automatic movements we have been unpacking with mindful attention in previous chapters, there are automatic habits of mind that you have been practising over and over again throughout your life. As a result, these habits have created neural networks in the brain that are smooth, fast, rapidly triggered and run automatically. In contrast, a new habit requires us to create a new neural pathway. This is effortful, slow, hard work, and requires your full attention.

It's possible you might get disheartened at first when you see how much these habits influence your behaviour. Seeing them for what they really are is the first step to changing a pattern. The old mental habits

*A new habit requires us to create a new neural pathway. This is effortful, slow, hard work, and requires your full attention.*

# Let's practise: holding the ball

'Holding the Ball' (also called 'Standing Stake') is a classic chi kung exercise, which explores, through your body, the habits that reveal themselves when you're faced with mild to moderate physical discomfort. It is highly likely that the way you deal with physical discomfort is similar to how you respond to mental discomfort.

Throughout this exercise make your breath the object of your attention. Breathe in through your nose and out through your mouth, using intention to breathe down both arms to your fingertips. Don't forget to keep breathing throughout – pay attention and notice if you start to hold your breath at any point.

① Begin in the tai chi standing posture (see page 36).

② Position your arms as if you are holding a big ball in front of your body, or as if you are hugging a tree.

③ Raise your arms up to roughly chest height with your fingers pointing toward each other. Face your palms toward your chest and keep your elbows more relaxed and pointing to the floor (a slightly harder version is to keep your elbows slightly bent and elevated to be in line with your wrists – try both). Bend your knees so that you sink into the pose, tucking the pelvis under and hollowing the chest slightly.

④ Hold this posture for as long as you can – aiming for at least 3 minutes the first time you practise. Be mindful about what happens as you keep your arms around the imaginary ball. Keep breathing.

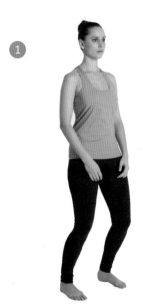
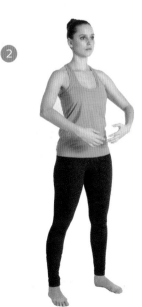
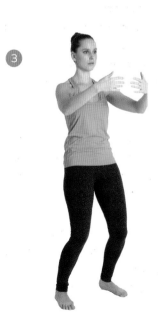

# holding the ball (continued)

⑤ In this posture, check yourself to see if you're frowning (if you are, you're likely straining your mind, too). Mindfully relax your face. Play around with having your eyes open and closed. You don't need to exert any effort with your eyes.

⑥ Remaining in the posture, and still breathing, deliberately focus your attention on specific body parts. Then, broaden your attention to encompass your whole body. Take your mind to the soles of your feet. Is your attention in your body or your mind?

⑦ Keep holding the posture. Keep breathing. What happens when you start to feel discomfort? How do your mind and body interact? At one moment your body is in your mind and you are observing sensations and working with your body, and the next minute your mind might wander either to an internal struggle or doubt, or to an external distraction. Pay attention to any thoughts in your mind that are related to moving or changing your posture – such as a sudden urge to scratch, or shift your weight. When your 3 minutes are up, or sooner if you have to, release your stance.

⑧ Consider how you felt during this exercise. You may have begun to notice tiredness and fatigue in your body. Your arms or shoulders or the top of your back may have begun to ache. What did your mind do with these sensations? Did it struggle against them? What did it feel like in your mind to have a direct experience of wanting things to be different? This exercise can help you to understand more about the types of habits that show themselves when something happens that you don't want, or you wish something were different. You're likely to meet these habits all the time in your daily life, so understanding what they look and feel like in your body is essential to your mindfulness training. Now, when you catch them, you can give them a quick label, before pausing, going into your body and checking out what the reaction is really all about.

Mindfully relax your face.

Take your focus down to the soles of your feet.

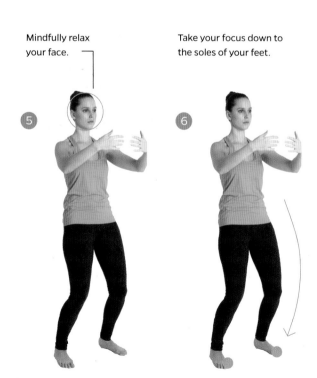

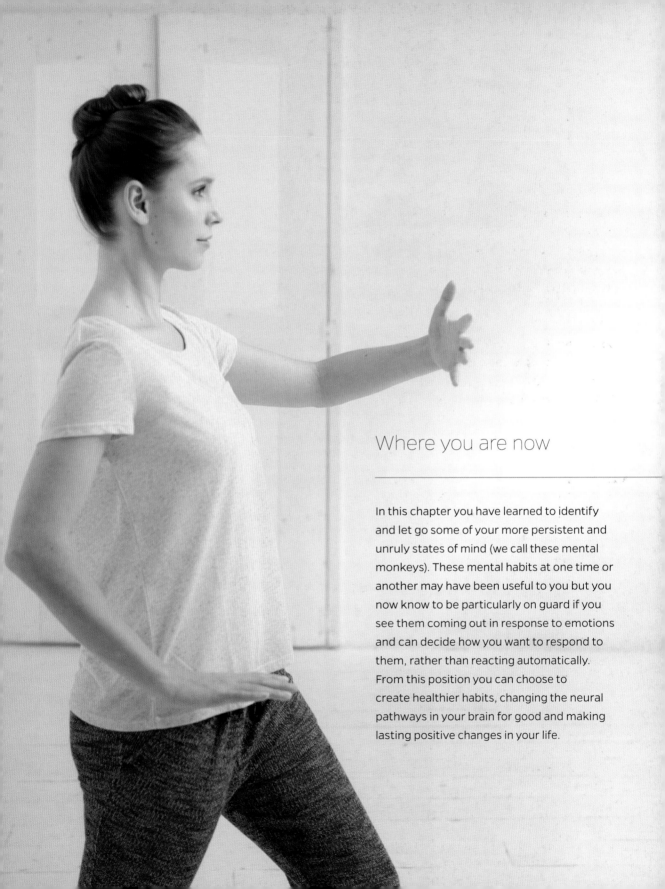

## Where you are now

In this chapter you have learned to identify and let go some of your more persistent and unruly states of mind (we call these mental monkeys). These mental habits at one time or another may have been useful to you but you now know to be particularly on guard if you see them coming out in response to emotions and can decide how you want to respond to them, rather than reacting automatically. From this position you can choose to create healthier habits, changing the neural pathways in your brain for good and making lasting positive changes in your life.

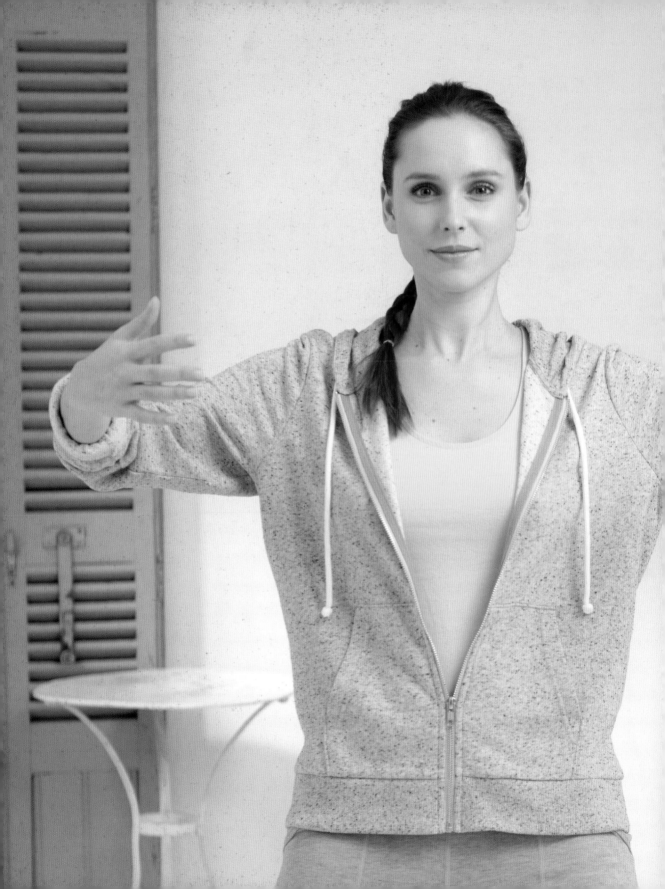

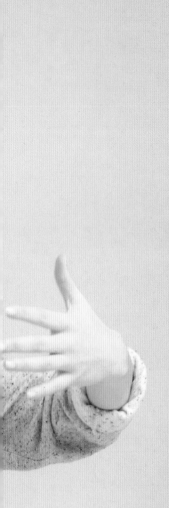

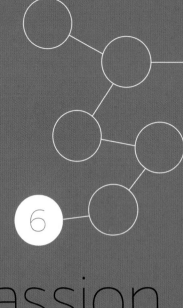

6

# Compassion

And so we reach the heart of the matter. After pausing, setting intentions and training our attention, we have gained some awareness of our monkey visitors and unhelpful mental habits. And every time we meet a thought, memory, image or bodily sensation and are able to greet it with acceptance and a smile, before bringing our mind back to the present moment, we are practising self-compassion.

Compassion is a wish to reduce suffering. Research has proven that self-compassion training can have a profoundly positive effect on our lives, helping us to build more nurturing, more sustainable habits. Showing ourselves compassion helps us to stop wasting valuable brain energy struggling against difficult mental experiences, and frees up space in our minds for creative and life-enhancing activities. The more self-compassionate we are, the better we feel!

# Welcoming emotions

Every time you are able to engage with and embrace difficult mental or physical experiences, you are caring for your emotions. This means you accept both the good and the bad – welcoming them equally, ideally with a smile.

T he process of turning toward the parts of ourselves that are difficult, painful and even ugly helps us to develop a new inner strength, enabling us to experience more joy and happiness in our lives. We no longer waste valuable brain energy trying to suppress, deny or avoid all the thoughts, feelings and emotions we have labelled as negative.

Research on the benefits of mindfulness shows that improvements in managing depression and anxiety are directly related to increased self-compassion.[1] Work with healthcare professionals also tells us that stress reduction is related to learning to be kind to ourselves.[2] This process of being kind to ourselves is often not easy at first – we are often our harshest critic and our own worst enemy. However, the more you practise engaging with all your sensations and emotions, both good and bad, the easier self-compassion becomes.

## Self-compassion saves brain energy

Endless mental struggle is exhausting. Each thought you have creates electrical and chemical activity in your brain. And, although your brain accounts for only 2 per cent of your bodyweight, it consumes 20 per cent of your total energy. Endless ruminating may seem like a way to avoid or fight negative or

Have a go

### Creativity as a route to self-acceptance

One way in which we can start to explore our emotions is through engagement with the creative arts. Art, poetry, music and dance can provoke different emotions and reactions within us, allowing us to observe parts of ourselves that we may not usually see. Be mindful how you respond to these arts, aware of how the body and mind react to works that you 'like' and 'don't like'. Remain curious and non-judgmental (or spot those judging monkeys as quickly as possible).

In his poem 'The Guest House', the Sufi poet Rumi captures the ethos of facing and accepting the challenging parts of ourselves in order to derive inner strength and joy. You'll find this and lots of other mindfulness poems online.[3] Which ones speak to you? Have someone read your favourites to you, so you can stay connected to your bodily experience as you absorb the words.

You can also try to write your own poetry to help you explore your mental and physical landscapes. A side-effect of mindfulness training is often the emergence of poems; students in mindfulness classes tend to write more of these as their training progresses.

## Brain training recap

With practice your mind will wander less and you'll be less distracted by mental chatter. Your brain will consume less energy, and you'll experience a huge sense of relief and relaxation in the space of the mind. Remember, though, that to release this energy, you have to put effort into regular mindfulness training. Only then will you become skilled at using your brain's resources more efficiently. When you notice your mind wandering into planning, analysing or judging (or any of our mental monkeys, see page 110–111), engage compassionately with your thoughts, accept them and let them go. When I find my own mind straying off the path, I try to remember 'free hugs'. These help me acknowledge what is going on in my mind, give whatever is there a hug, and then quickly release it without attaching to it in any way. Then, I return to the raw sensations of my body. The earlier I notice my mind wandering, the sooner I can give my free hug and let go, stepping back into the 'now'.

difficult experiences, but in fact a more effective response is to stop running away or fighting, and to turn *toward* what you fear. Although this may sound like a crazy suggestion, facing your fear and accepting it means that fear and negativity begin to dissipate. Then, you can begin truly to liberate your mind.

In the illustration below, the black arrows show you how much brain energy endless thinking – worrying, ruminating, rehearsing – uses up. Mindfulness allows you to recall your mind to the 'now'.

In this chapter I'll explore self-compassion in more detail through carefully designed BMT exercises that help you to develop your capacity for compassion through mindfulness of the body. With training, you can increase your ability to stay with bodily and mental sensations, a critical part of the compassion-training process. You'll discover how the route to compassion starts with a full awareness of non-compassion, training in accepting difficult thoughts and feelings before bringing the mind back to the present moment. You'll learn how to use your brain's energy resources more efficiently by switching from a default mode of fear-oriented withdrawal to a more spacious, open attitude toward life and living.

## Recalling the mind

The black dots indicate anxious thoughts; the red dot (in 1) is the moment of mindfulness, bringing the mind back to the 'now'. A moment of compassion (hearts, in 2) also brings us back to the 'now'; with training this can happen ever more quickly in the mind-wandering process.

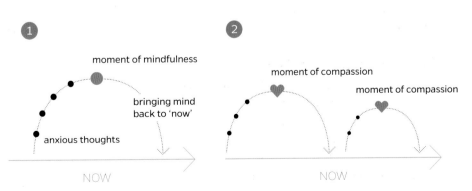

# Acknowledging difficult thoughts

There may be some thoughts that you are not ready to embrace fully – and this is where the really interesting work begins.

I realize that so far it sounds a little too easy. Inevitably, there will be some physical or mental states that seem too difficult or painful to delve into, or some entrenched habits that have been with you for so many years it's not easy to let them go and learn to love yourself fully.

When these stickier thoughts appear, you may find that your instinct is to get frustrated with yourself and angry with your practice – after all, you've been working hard at staying mindful, so how can you still be making mistakes? This is the judging monkey coming out in full force. Beware – often this monkey is so quick to emerge and take over that you may not see it coming, allowing it rapidly to get out of hand. You might even notice you are judging the fact you are judging!

When you notice a habit that you can't drop immediately, you can still be mindful. Rather than feeling frustrated at this point, try to feel grateful and inspired that you have actually spotted the

habit – this is progress! It's also a great opportunity to pause and be kind to yourself. Be patient, do your best to let go of any secondary judging, and perhaps make a commitment to work with the primary habit when you're ready.

Eventually, with practice, your whole approach to life can become more compassionate. You may start to notice how you are not just responding to thoughts and feelings compassionately as they arise, but you're actually living in a more naturally compassionate mind state.

## Awareness of non-compassion

You might observe as you do this training that at first you become more aware of those states of mind you are actually seeking to let go of. Similarly, your route to compassion, kindness and acceptance often initially arises from a growing awareness of those times when you are *not* being kind to yourself or others.

Although I am not a Buddhist, occasionally I attend Buddhist retreats and courses to deepen my mindfulness practice. One Easter, I signed up for a weekend compassion retreat as a special treat, an act of self-care. What I actually experienced, however, completely shocked me. During the

When we engage compassionately with our emotions, the compassion magnet draws out its opposite – all that is non-compassion.

retreat I became aware of the most intense, vivid and violent fantasies, and between the practice sessions all I could do was curl up in a ball and sleep.

I realized that my exhaustion was the result of my struggle against the parts of myself that I didn't want to accept or engage with. An American Insight Meditation teacher, Andrea Fella,[4] whose work I draw on frequently, helped me to really understand what had happened here. She describes compassion as a magnet. When we engage compassionately with our emotions, the compassion magnet draws out its opposite – all that is non-compassion. This is the stuff we have to work through.

This is the challenge as we go deeper into mindfulness. Being compassionate and mindful with all the nice stuff is the easy bit. It's when we meet the difficult parts with kindness and acceptance (non-judging) that we can really make progress.

## Compassion and courage

Buddhists use the phrase 'invite Mara for tea' to illustrate openness toward the difficult. The Taoists call it 'jumping into the dragon's mouth', which captures the courage necessary in this process. Facing these fears is what will set us free. I am constantly grateful to all the clients I have worked with over the years who have inspired me with their tremendous courage as they engage with really difficult emotional material.

> Compassionate engagement with emotions, even the difficult ones, is part of Buddhist practice.

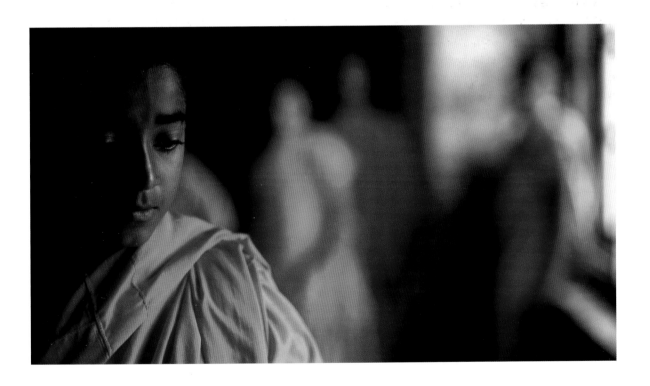

# Creating space in your mind

When you can spot and drop mind-wandering more quickly, you create space in your mind. The antics of your mental monkeys no longer consume so much energy, meaning you have more of it. Cultivating acceptance is the key to releasing this energy for the things in life that really matter.

Trying to get away from negative experiences leads us into cycles of reactivity (thinking and struggle). When this happens the whole mind–body system constricts. This narrowed focus becomes our whole reality, we lose perspective, and are less able to consider the world around us. This is your brain in 'it's all about me' mode (see page 114). At this point you need to reverse the constriction, open up your focus and create more space in your mind.

In 'Go Big', the exercise on pages 127–9, you'll practise staying with difficult experiences and observing all the tricks your mind plays when you try to reverse mental constriction. This perspective will allow you to see things more clearly. Keep in mind that your main intention is to be kind to yourself no matter what you experience.

The key point to remember here is that when we accept what is going on, by dropping judgment and attempts at managing experience, we save brain energy. Although it sounds easy, in practice is can be more of a challenge. It's also important to remember that we are not just passively accepting things that we experience. We are accepting them by paying attention, on purpose and with a commitment to grow and develop ourselves.

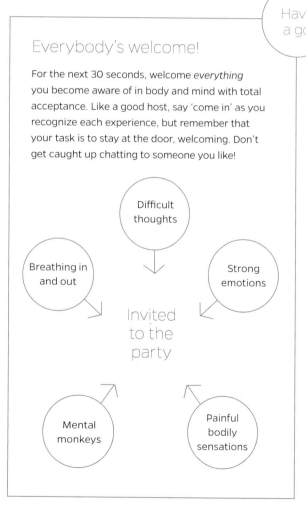

Have a go

## Everybody's welcome!

For the next 30 seconds, welcome *everything* you become aware of in body and mind with total acceptance. Like a good host, say 'come in' as you recognize each experience, but remember that your task is to stay at the door, welcoming. Don't get caught up chatting to someone you like!

Difficult thoughts

Breathing in and out

Strong emotions

Invited to the party

Mental monkeys

Painful bodily sensations

# Let's practise:
# go big

This exercise works well as part of your regular practice, especially if you have a recurring issue that raises negative emotions within you. Equally, though, if you are reacting to a single incident (such as a particularly frustrating commute, or when you're in the thick of a strong emotion during a heated argument), it provides an instant opportunity to accept the emotions that occur. Stay directly with your bodily sensations throughout the exercise. The mental monkeys will come out for sure, but remember that they are welcome – just go big with them to reduce their power and come back to the raw sensations of your body. Remember, you are learning a skill. Be kind to yourself and start with the mild to moderate sensations at first, building up your confidence so that you are ready to use the technique during times of high stress. Practise the exercise in a quiet environment initially. At the start you'll move your arms, but once you've really grasped the concept of expanding your thinking, you can use small movements with your hands or just make the movement in your mind. The body movements represent the movement you are trying to make with your mind. Arms lifting up, to allow the full emotion to arise; arms opening to create maximum space to really feel the emotion; and arms closing in a hugging movement, indicating your desire to welcome, to embrace your experience, no matter what.

① Begin in the tai chi standing posture (see page 36), connecting to the raw sensations of your body. Bring to mind a mildly difficult situation that has been troubling you (such as managing a difficult boss), one that provokes a mild degree of emotional reactivity or discomfort in your body. Resist the urge to pick the most challenging thing in your life (although you can work up to this).

② Engage with your bodily sensations as you deliberately generate thoughts, images and memories about the situation. Be curious about the sensations, becoming particularly aware of any movement through the region of your torso. Notice how you split your attention between generating the content and observing the bodily and mental response to it.

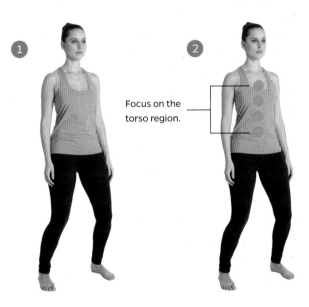

Focus on the torso region.

# go big
# (continued)

③ As you start to raise your arms, use your body to help your mind understand what you want it to do – literally to expand, to go big, to arise as much as it needs to.

④ As the feeling is allowed to arise, gently begin to open your arms so that you experience all the feeling without constraining it. Create space for your emotion by opening your arms far out to the sides. As you do so, squeeze your shoulderblades together, opening your chest.

⑤ As your arms move apart, create a big space in your mind around the emotion. This mental space indicates you are willing to accept all the emotions related to your chosen situation – none gets preferential treatment, none is denied. Your mental space is saying 'my mind is big enough to hold all of this; don't be afraid'.

⑥ Within this large open arm movement not only have you created space for your emotion, but also for the sensations of your feet on the floor, the sensations of your breath, the sensation of the sun on your skin, the sensations of your clothes. They are all there, all welcome, and all given equal billing.

⑦ Now, reverse the movement, bringing your arms back together, fingers pointing toward each other. Create a slight roundedness in your back.

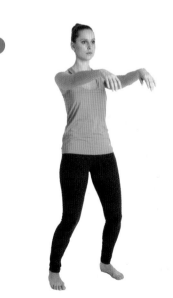

3

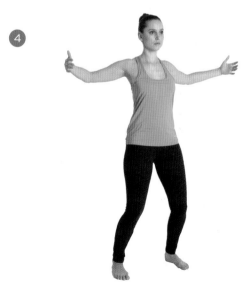

4

In this movement you are hugging your difficult emotion, bringing it close to you, genuinely accepting, embracing and acknowledging all of it.

⑧ On your next out-breath, anchor your attention into your body and allow your arms to return to the starting position. Repeat the whole process as many times as you need to give your emotions enough space to fully unfold. It might take five to ten repetitions to feel fully at ease. Pause and rest your mind in the body for a moment. You can use the Mindfulness of the Soles of the Feet exercise (see page 96) to ground yourself if needed.

Taking it further

## Deeper levels of practice

The ego (or self) and the habits it has developed to protect itself can react very strongly when we start to manage it differently. If we have a genuine wish to connect to a deeper, more spiritual aspect of the self, then there's no alternative but to move through the ego's strong reactions. Moving beyond ego reveals to us our connection to all living things.

With extended practice you may experience a state of mind referred to as *ru ding* or 'fear of the death of the ego'.[5] Taoist master Bruce Frantzis describes this as 'an amorphous, nonspecific fear [which] paralyses you right down to the centre of your being, pervading every cell of your body and every crevice of your mind'. Don't panic, you will survive!

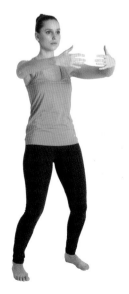

7

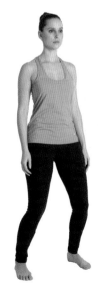

8

# Compassion in culture

Mindfulness in motion helps you to practise compassion in your daily life. Attending to your body, mind, emotions and reactions reverses the damaging effects of our technology-oriented, highly distracted, often disembodied ways of living.

C ompassion – for the self and for others – is central to traditional Eastern practices such as tai chi and chi kung, but conditions in the modern world seem to optimize non-compassionate states of mind. In tai chi the phrase *wu wei* describes a type of non-action that is in itself action; it is doing in non-doing. This is what we aspire to when faced with difficult situations. Non-doing involves honestly engaging with our own feelings, whatever they are, in that moment, and attending deeply to our body. This is not only an act of kindness to ourselves, but it's the way we genuinely connect with others.

This contagious element of mindfulness is important. What others see makes them curious, supports them to value their own body and mind, and gives them the courage to try something different, too. I often see this contagion when I'm teaching in open spaces in London. People stop and observe my students as they are mindfully walking or engaging with nature and it makes them wonder (and often mimic) what we are doing.

## Compassion in a modern world

We live in a world dominated by fear and uncertainty. Since getting rid of my TV, I am more alert to how

## The practice

### Self-compassion is contagious

One nurse who attended a BMT course set the broad intention to be kinder to herself during her working day. She would usually skip lunch (even on a long shift), prioritizing paperwork and the needs of the patients over herself, but this time she decided to pause, and to take the time to eat. This small act of self-compassion, just 15 minutes out of the day for herself, had a huge impact on the rest of her day. Having valued herself in this small way, she was able to connect with others with an openness and engagement that meant she worked more effectively. Not only that, there was a ripple effect among her colleagues. Other staff became curious about this 'rebel' who against prevailing culture was showing care to herself. This gave them their own courage to think that they too deserved to stop and eat.

quickly these emotions can rise in me. Now, when I find myself watching the news, I am acutely aware of the change in my body – a tightening or tensing, an increase in my heart rate, and a sense of unease. Repeated engagement with (and suppression of) low-level but chronic stressors like these numbs our emotional sensitivity. I didn't realize until I stopped watching the news what an impact it had on my emotional state. Think of our young people, growing up with never-ending commentary on the financial crisis, limited job opportunities and global warming.

One way of coping with all of this fear is to disconnect from the body, to ignore or turn away from the feelings as they arise within us. Studies show that one consequence of this attitude is escalating rates of childhood mental health conditions and addiction. (Training our young people in compassion and mindfulness of the body is an urgent priority.)

In the modern world we are also more susceptible to the musculoskeletal problems arising from working with laptops, mobile phones, tablets and innumerable other mobile devices. Under these conditions, our bodies suffer from the strain of awkward postures and constant mental agitation. They might cry out in pain – but in order to keep going, keep pushing forward, we ignore the cries.

Ignoring the body is not only bad for our own mental and physical health, it also fundamentally reduces our ability to connect with others. If we can't acknowledge our own pain, how can we have the space in our lives to acknowledge that of others?

> We need to find the time in our demanding schedules to be kind to ourselves, to reconnect with our bodies and with nature.

Have a go

## Just like me

Mimic someone walking down the street, as you did in the exercise in Chapter 3 (see page 68). Stay connected to your body and mind as you do so, and each time you notice a thought, image or bodily sensation arise, say to yourself 'Just like me, perhaps this person has felt pain' or 'Just like me, perhaps this person heard the sound of the bus' or 'Just like me, perhaps this person has felt anger, loneliness, boredom' and so on. Whatever you feel or experience, as you mimic the walk, imagine that the person you are mimicking feels or experiences 'just like you'.

The exercise serves to remind us that all people have feelings, emotions and physical pain that they might act on in unskilful ways – just like you do, or I do. In itself, this helps us connect to our powers of empathy – to feel compassion.

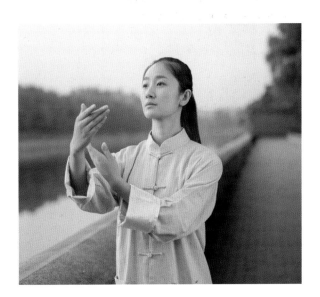

# Compassion in the brain

To develop compassion we must stay engaged with our own emotional life through our bodies. If you keep your body in mind, and learn about those brain regions that code for your movement and your emotions, you'll be well on your way.

In the last topic you learned how to put yourself in someone else's shoes by mimicking that person's walk. To develop compassion it is vital to experience through the body the whole breadth of our emotional life. This will help us to understand directly that what we feel is the same as what others feel. Brain-imaging studies with monks who specialize in compassionate mind meditation reveal that human beings do not use their fancy frontal lobes – the thinking, planning, analysing brain regions – to generate compassion.[6] When provoked to experience emotions, the monks showed greater activity in the right anterior insula and somatosensory cortex. These findings suggest that there may be greater sensitivity, specificity and subtlety in the awareness of body and emotional states with compassionate mind training. These are the regions related to processing signals from the body – the exact areas we work with in BMT.

We met the insula in the previous chapter where connections between this structure and different

## Effects of compassionate mind training

The somatosensory cortex processes all the sensations from the body; more of this region is dedicated to hands and face than any other body part (see page 79). The right insula cortex processes the slightly more abstract sense of emotions that move through the body. Both these regions were found to be more active in research on monks specializing in compassionate meditation.

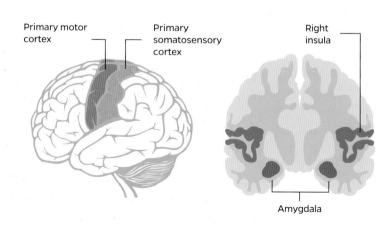

Primary motor cortex

Primary somatosensory cortex

Right insula

Amygdala

SURFACE OF BRAIN

SLICE VIEW OF BRAIN

parts of the frontal cortex determined whether the emotion we feel is an overwhelming 'It's all about me' experience, or just one of many sensations that make up the contents of the moment-by-moment mindscape. This densely connected area has fingers in many pies as it's linked to the somatosensory and motor cortices, various parts of the frontal and temporal lobes, and other brain regions. When we train in mindfulness, the size of this structure increases (particularly on the right side of the brain)[7] – mindfulness quite literally grows this part of the brain.

The insula (and also the anterior cingulate – a part of the attention network, see page 77) is also home to some special neurons called Von Economo neurons.[8] The size and shape of these neurons suggest that their job is to send electrical signals quickly over large distances, co-ordinating emotion, action and awareness. They play an important role in socially relevant situations, including the processing of positive and negative emotions, and empathy. They are found in humans and great apes, and, intriguingly, also in elephants and whales – two species known for their highly sophisticated (if little-understood) social structures and complex emotional lives.

Von Economo neurons are more prominent on the right side of the brain and relate to our ability to exert effortful attentional control even in the face of strong emotions. This is at the heart of mindfulness training.

## Free your right hemisphere

Fighting with your emotions uses up valuable energy in the right hemisphere of your brain. The right side is our ticket to survival, as it engages us in activities that can quickly get us away from danger – we need this if a tiger is about to attack us, but it's redundant if our anxiety is triggered by such things as fear of rejection, judgment, uncertainty or other socially conditioned fears that will not physically harm us.

Activity in the right brain is associated with arousal, aversion, avoidance and individual-oriented (survival) emotions. But what can happen if we turn to embrace and engage with these emotions? What happens when we face our fears and no longer expend so much right-brain energy on dealing with them? One suggestion is that this might free up the right hemisphere's other functions, which include engaging with the world with a broad openness to whatever might be there, without any need to know the outcome, thus supporting creativity and innovation.[9] Remember we can also access this state of mind via deliberate engagement with creative arts (see page 122).

With mindfulness training we learn to engage with all our experiences, increasing our capacity to feel positive and compassionate more of the time.

## Loving kindness

Now for the culmination of all your training. Loving kindness is just one of four compassionate meditation trainings in Buddhism. Known collectively as the Four Immeasurables, they comprise equanimity, empathic joy, loving kindness and compassion. When we train in loving kindness, we boost the compassion network in the brain. The loving kindness exercise on pages 134–5 asks you to think about a loved one to deliberately generate bodily sensations, and then turns up these sensations to create a deep, heartfelt desire and wish for all beings to be free from suffering.

# Let's practise: loving kindness

The exercise combines both loving kindness (a wish for yourself and others to be happy) as well as compassion (a wish for diminished suffering). Practise it with a close attention to raw bodily sensations – which allows you to really experience heartfelt desire in your body. While you're learning, practise in a quiet space. Then, as you get more adept, practise while you're on the go, any time and anywhere. The exercise will give you a sense of how your body engages or disengages with compassion. Practise it often, as your experience will be different every time you have a go. You don't have to work with the same people each time (see below), but it might help to be consistent while you're still learning. Think of yourself as a scientist. It helps to have some method in your explorations.

## Common responses

People connect with the Loving Kindness exercise in very different ways. Some struggle to have any feeling at all. If that's you, that's okay – just keep practising, being sure to embrace any judging such as 'I can't do this' or 'I am not good enough' and, most of all, maintain your curiosity.

Some are surprised by the strength of their feelings either for the loved or the difficult person. In level 3 (your difficult person), you may find it painful to really open up and allow your feelings space. You may even become tearful. Be kind to yourself and embrace all your experience. The phrase 'this too will pass' or remembering to 'go big' (see page 127) might be helpful here.

① Sit comfortably, in a place where you will not be disturbed. Bring to mind someone in your life who makes you smile, or a much-loved pet. Thinking of this person (or pet) creates a warm feeling in your torso. Use mindfulness of your face and body to connect to the sensations. Feel your torso (and the heart region). Attend to your hands and face.

② Try to 'ramp up' your image of this person (or pet), with details such as their voice, their smell, the places you saw them. Be mindful of any sensations in your torso as you bring these memories to mind and increase the vividness of these mental experiences.

③ Stay with your feelings – use effort to 'turn up the volume' and maintain your sense of love, kindness, warmth – whatever positive emotions you are feeling at this time, in your body. (Take care not to get lost

## Levels of compassion

In BMT we give each category of person in this exercise a 'level'. These are the levels we use.

**Level 1** – someone who makes you smile
**Level 2** – someone who is neutral
**Level 3** – someone who is difficult
**Level 4** – yourself
**Level 5** – everyone in levels 1–4

in imagery and memory – you are just using these as tools to generate the bodily sensation. You might be aware that you are switching attention between head and heart in this practice. That's okay for now.)

④ Keeping the image of your chosen person in mind and, staying directly connected to your bodily sensations, repeat the following phrases in your head three times (or make up your own if you wish):

**May you be safe and protected**
**May you be healthy**
**May you live at peace and with kindness**

⑤ Now start thinking about a neutral person. This is someone whom you might see every day, but don't know personally; someone whose image you can generate reliably, but who doesn't have a strong emotional attachment for you. (Your local shopkeeper is a good example.) Repeat steps 1 to 4.

⑥ Repeat steps 1 to 4 again, but this time for someone in your life with whom you have issues, such as a challenging work colleague or someone who has recently criticized or upset you. Pay special attention to your hands and face, where more subtle aspects of our emotional state can emerge.

⑦ Repeat steps 1 to 4, this time for yourself. Be alert to mental movements (such as sudden tiredness, boredom or switching off) and renew your intention to stay directly with your bodily sensations.

⑧ Finally, widen the circle of compassion and repeat steps 1 to 4 to include everyone you've chosen. 'Just like me' they all have the desire to be happy and free from suffering.

⑨ Now consider your responses in this exercise. How did the sensations in your body change (or not) when you went from the person who makes you smile to the neutral person? What was similar or different in your mental and physical response as you changed levels (see box, opposite)? What did you notice about the way you selected individuals for each level? Did any mental monkeys appear when you confronted a difficult person or yourself? What did your mind do when you got to yourself? What happened when you combined everyone together?

Taking it further

## Be your most difficult person

Turning toward yourself can be the most difficult part of this exercise. Your mind may start to wander or you might become very sleepy. Be curious, notice how your mind is easily distracted when faced with strong emotions or discomfort, particularly when you try to generate compassion for yourself. (Interestingly, when this exercise first came to the West from Eastern practices, instructors asked their students to begin with themselves and work outward. Westerners found this too difficult – so the order was reversed.)

# All about us

There are many aspects of modern life that hamper our ability to be compassionate. However, your practice has shown you that even tiny changes to the way you treat yourself can have surprising ripple effects on those around you.

Training ourselves to stay directly with our bodily experience as we generate compassionate thoughts and feelings energizes our insula – changing a whole network of brain regions responsible for emotional regulation, compassion and empathy. In turn, as we acknowledge our own suffering and are compassionate toward it, we are able to feel more empathy for others, increasing our connection to the whole of humanity. At this point life becomes less 'all about me' and more 'all about us' – a switch that has a profound effect on the health and wellbeing of our society as a whole.

Now all that remains is for you to keep on practising. Above all, never give up. You will likely experience moments of doubt along the way, times when it all seems like too much effort, when you are tempted to give up and go back to your old unhelpful ways of thinking and behaving. In these moments, simply pause and take heart – this is all a necessary part of the learning process. Just remind yourself how far you have come, and carry on. Always be kind to yourself. While the journey won't always be easy, it cannot fail to be rewarding. Every step that you take along the mindfulness path brings you closer to lasting peace and happiness, true freedom of mind.

> The smallest of mindful actions can have a ripple effect on those around you.

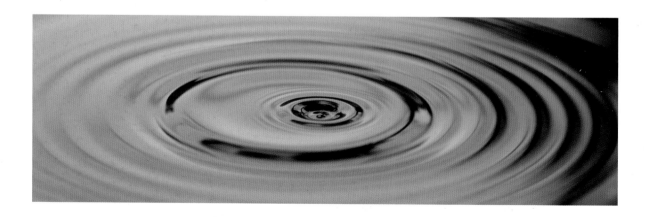

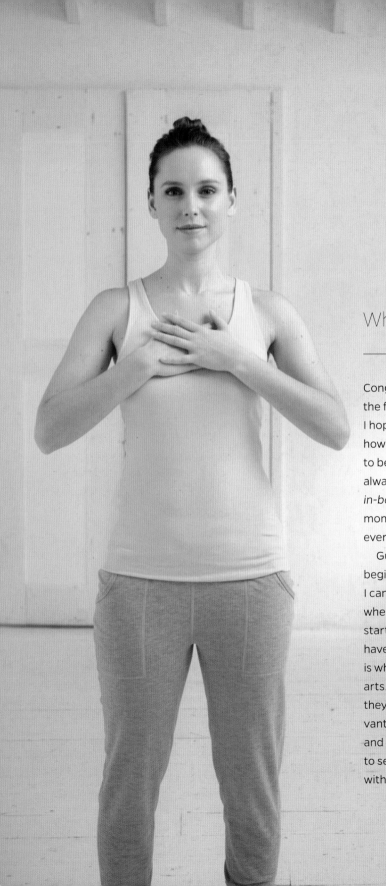

## Where you are now

Congratulations! You have now completed
the first stage of your mindfulness training.
I hope this guide has given you a taste for
how different things can be when you dare
to be more present in your life. Remember,
always keep the *body-in-mind* and the *mind-in-body*. Your body is your key to the present
moment, and the present moment is all you
ever truly have.

  Guess what? It's time to go back to the
beginning! If you have done the exercises,
I can guarantee you that the mind you had
when you engaged with the material at the
start of this book is not the same mind you
have now. Going back to the beginners' class
is what we do with all black belts in martial
arts. Not only do they get a real surprise as
they revisit the basic exercises from a new
vantage point, often finding much richness
and depth as a result, they also have a chance
to see whether they can continue to engage
with the curious eyes of a child. Good luck!

# Notes

## Introduction

**1** Rosch, E, Thompson, E and Varela, F J (1992). *The Embodied Mind: Cognitive Science and Human Experience*. MIT Press.

**2** Kerr, C E, Sacchet, M D, Lazar, S W, Moore, C I and Jones, S R (2013). Mindfulness starts with the body: Somatosensory attention and top-down modulation of cortical alpha rhythms in mindfulness meditation. *Frontiers in Human Neuroscience*, 7, 12, 1–15.

**3** Michalak, J, Rohde, K, and Troje, N F (2014). How we walk affects what we remember: Gait modifications through biofeedback change negative affective memory bias. *Journal of Behavior Therapy and Experimental Psychiatry* 46, 121–125.

**4** Grepmair, L, Mitterlehner, F, Loew, T, Bachler, E, Rother, W, and Nickel, M (2007). Promoting mindfulness in psychotherapists in training influences the treatment results of their patients: A randomized, double-blind, controlled study. *Psychotherapy and Psychosomatics.* 76, 332–338.

Keane, A (2013). The influence of therapist mindfulness practice on psychotherapeutic work: A mixed-methods study. *Mindfulness (N Y)*, 689–703.

**5** Russell, T A, Green, M and Coltheart, M (2008). Remediation of facial emotion perception: Concomitant changes in visual attention. *Schizophrenia Research*, 103 (1-3), 248–256.

Marsh, P J, Luckett, G, Russell, T A, Coltheart, M and Green, M J (2012). Effects of facial emotion recognition remediation on visual scanning of novel face stimuli. *Schizophrenia Research*, 141 (2-3), 234-40.

Marsh, P, Green, M J, Russell, T A, McGuire, J, Harris, A and Coltheart, M (2010). Remediation of facial emotion recognition in schizophrenia: Functional predictors, generalizability, and durability. *American Journal of Psychiatric Rehabilitation*, 13 (2), 143–170.

**6** Grossman, P, Niemann, L, Schmidt, S and Walach, H (2004). Mindfulness-based stress reduction and health benefits: A meta-analysis. *Journal of Psychosomatic Research*, 57, 35–43.

Williams, M and Kuyken, W (2012). Mindfulness-based cognitive therapy: A promising new approach to preventing depressive relapse. *British Journal of Psychiatry*, 200, 359–360.

Khoury, B, Lecomte, T, Fortin, G, Masse, M, Therien, P, Bouchard, V, Chapleau, M-A, Paquin, K and Hofmann, S (2013). Mindfulness-based therapy: A comprehensive meta-analysis. *Clinical Psychology Review*, 33, 763–77.

**7** Hölzel, B K, Lazar, S W, Gard, T, Schuman-Olivier, Z, Vago, D R and Ott, U (2011). How does mindfulness meditation work? Proposing mechanisms of action from a conceptual and neural perspective. *Perspectives on Psychological Science*, 6 (6), 37–559.

Carmody, J and Baer, R (2008). Relationships between mindfulness practice and levels of mindfulness, medical and psychological symptoms and well-being in a mindfulness-based stress reduction program. *Journal of Behavioural Medicine*, 31 (1), 23–33.

**8** Russell, T A (2011). Body In Mind Training: Mindful movement for severe and enduring mental illness. *British Journal of Wellbeing*, 2 (3), 13–16.

**9** Russell, T A and Tatton-Ramos, T P (2014). Body In Mind Training: Mindful movement for the clinical setting. *Neuro-Disability and Psychotherapy*, 2 (1/2), 108–136.

**10** Kabat-Zinn, J (2003). Mindfulness-based interventions in context: Past, present, and future. *Clinical Psychology: Science and Practice*, 10 (2), 144–156.

**11** Russell, T A (2011).

Russell, T A and Arcuri S A (2015). A neurophysiological and neuropsychological consideration of mindful movement. *Frontiers in Human Neuroscience*. 8.

**12** King, E (2011). A Modified MBCT Program for employed people with bipolar disorder. MSc Dissertation, Mental Health Studies, King's College London, Institute of Psychiatry.

Wong, M (2011). The effects of mindfulness-based cognitive therapy on psychosocial functioning in employed bipolar patients. MSc Dissertation, Mental Health Studies, King's College London, Institute of Psychiatry.

Bland, D (2013). Does mindfulness training improve body awareness in naïve mindfulness practitioners? MSc Dissertation, Neuroscience, King's College London, Institute of Psychiatry.

## Chapter 1

**1** Kerr, C E, Sacchet, M D, Lazar, S W, Moore, C I and Jones, S R (2013). Mindfulness starts with the body: Somatosensory attention and top-down modulation of cortical alpha rhythms in mindfulness meditation. *Frontiers in Human Neuroscience*, 7, 12, 1–15.

**2** Hay, D B, Williams, D, Stahl, D and Wingate, R J (2013). Using drawings of the brain cell to exhibit expertise in neuroscience: Exploring the boundaries of experimental culture. *Science Education*, 97 (3), 468–491.

**3** Goleman, D, Kabat-Zinn J and Tan, C M (2012). *Search Inside Yourself: Increase Productivity, Creativity and Happiness*. Harper Collins.

**4** Grossman, P, Niemann, L, Schmidt, S, and Walach, H (2004). Mindfulness-based stress reduction and health benefits. A meta-analysis. *Journal of Psychosomatic Research*, 57, 35–43.

Khoury, B, Lecomte, T, Fortin, G, Masse, M, Therien, P, Bouchard, V, Chapleau, M-A, Paquin, K and Hofmann, S (2013). Mindfulness-based therapy: A comprehensive meta-analysis. *Clinical Psychology Review*, 33, 763–771.

**5** Williams, M and Kuyken, W (2012). Mindfulness-based cognitive therapy: A promising new approach to preventing depressive relapse. *British Journal of Psychiatry*, 200, 359–360.

**6** Anderson, D I, Campos, J J, Witherington, D C, Dahl, A, Rivera, M, He, M, Uchiyama, I, Barbu-Roth, M and Poehlman, A T (2013). The role of locomotion in psychological development. *Frontiers in Psychology*, 4, 440, 1017.

**7** Hillman, C H, Erickson, K I and Kramer, A F (2008). Be smart, exercise your heart: Exercise effects on brain and cognition. *Nature Reviews Neuroscience*, 9 (1), 58–65.

**8** Hyde K L, Lerch J, Norton A, Forgeard M, Winner E, Evans A C, Schlaug G (2009). The effects of musical training on structural brain development: A longitudinal study. *Annals of the New York Academy of Sciences*, 1169, 182–6.

**9** Anderson, D I et al (2013).

**10** Wolpert, D (2011). TED Talk: 'The Real Reason for Brains'. At: www.ted.com/talks/daniel_wolpert_the_real_reason_for_brains?language=en

**11** Payne, P and Crane-Godreau, M A (2013). Meditative movement for depression and Anxiety. *Frontiers in Psychiatry*, 4, 71.

**12** Wilson, M (2002). Six views of embodied cognition. *Psychonomic Bulletin and Review*, 9 (4), 625-636.

**13** Rosch, E, Thompson, E and Varela, F J (1992). *The Embodied Mind: Cognitive Science and Human Experience*. MIT Press.

**14** Wallace, B A (2013). *Meditations of a Buddhist Sceptic: A Manifesto for the Mind Sciences*. Columbia University Press.

**15** www.mindandlife.org

**16** A great weblink for this is the YouTube clip 'Neuroplasticity' (Sentis): www.youtube.com/watch?v=ELpfYCZa87g

**17** Hölzel, B K, Lazar, S. W, Gard, T, Schuman-Olivier, Z, Vago, D R and Ott U (2011). How does mindfulness meditation work? Proposing mechanisms of action from a conceptual and neural perspective. *Perspectives on Psychological Science*, 6 (6), 537–559

**18** Dayan, E, and Cohen, L G (2011). Neuroplasticity subserving motor skill learning. *Neuron* 72, 443–54.

**19** Hölzel et al (2011)

## Chapter 2

**1** Kerr, C E, Sacchet, M D, Lazar, S W, Moore, C I and Jones, S R (2013). Mindfulness starts with the body: Somatosensory attention and top-down modulation of cortical alpha rhythms in mindfulness meditation. *Frontiers in Human Neuroscience*, 7, 12, 1–15.

See also Catherine Kerr on YouTube: www.youtube.com/watch?v=AGnGRgyLwMs

**2** Clayton, R B, Leshner, G and Almond, A (2015). The extended iSelf: The impact of iPhone separation on cognition, emotion, and physiology. *Journal of Computer-Mediated Communication*, 20 (2), 119-135.

**3** Berman, M, Jonides, J and Kaplan, S (2009). The cognitive benefits of interacting with nature. *Psychological Science*, 19, 1207–1212.

**4** Jha, A P, Krompinger, J and Baime, M J (2007). Mindfulness training modifies subsystems of attention. *Cognitive, Affective, and Behavioral Neuroscience*, 7 (2), 109-119.

**5** Salman, M S (2002). The cerebellum: it's about time! But timing is not everything – new insights into the role of the cerebellum in timing motor and cognitive tasks. *Journal of Child Neurology*, 17, 1–9.

**6** Rubia, K, Russell, T A, Overmeyer, S, Brammer, M J, Bullmore, E T, Sharma, T, Simmons, A, Williams, S C R, Giampietro, V, Andrew, C and Taylor, E (2001). Mapping motor inhibition: Generic brain activations across different versions of go-no-go and stop tasks. *NeuroImage*, 13 (2), 250–261. Quote from page 250.

**7** Li F, Harmer P, Fisher K J, McAuley E, Chaumeton N, Eckstrom E and Wilson N L (2005). Tai chi and fall reductions in older adults: A randomized controlled trial. *Journal of Gerontology*, 60A (2), 187–94.

**8** Dillon, D, and Pizzagalli, D (2012). Inhibition of action, thought, and emotion: A selective neurobiological review. *Applied and Preventative Psychology* 29, 997-10.

**9** Liverant, G I, Brown, T A, Barlow, D H and Roemer, L (2008). Emotion regulation in unipolar depression: The effects of acceptance and suppression of subjective emotional experience on the intensity and duration of sadness and negative affect. *Behaviour Research and Therapy*, 46 (11), 1201-1209.

**10** Berkman, E T, Burklund, L and Lieberman, M D (2009). Inhibitory spillover: Intentional motor inhibition produces incidental limbic inhibition via right inferior frontal cortex. *Neuroimage*, 47, 705–712.

**11** Kozasa, E, Sato, J, Lacerada, S, Barreiros, M, Radvany, J, Russell, T A, Sanches, L, Mello, L and Amaro, Jr, E (2012). Meditation training increased brain efficiency in an attention task. *Neuroimage*, 59, 745–749.

**12** Lieberman, M D (2009.) The brain's braking system (and how to 'use your words' to tap into it). *NeuroLeadership*, 2. At: www.neuroleadership.com/wp-content/uploads/2009/02/A1-TBBS-US.pdf

**13** Lieberman, M D, Eisenberger, N I, Crockett, M J, Tom, S, Pfeifer, J H, Way, B M (2007). Putting feelings into words: Affect labelling disrupts amygdala activity to affective stimuli. *Psychological Science*, 18, 421–428.

**14** Craig, A D (2009). How do you feel – now? The anterior insula and human awareness. *Nature Reviews Neuroscience*, 10, 59–70.

Paulus, M P and Stein, M B (2006). An insular view of anxiety. *Biological Psychiatry*, 60, 383–387.

**15** Luders, E, Kurth, F, Mayer, E A, Toga, A W, Narr, K L and Gaser, C (2012). The unique brain anatomy of meditation practitioners: Alterations in cortical gyrification. *Frontiers in Human Neuroscience*, 6, 1–9.

**16** Nummenmaa, L, Glerean, E, Hari, R and Hietanen, J (2014). Bodily maps of emotions. *Proceedings of the National Academy of Science*, 111 (2), 646–651.

**17** Meijer, M de (1989). The contribution of general features of body movement to the attribution of emotions. *Journal of Nonverbal Behavior*, 13 (4), 247–268.

**18** An online animation about mood and body movement: www.biomotionlab.ca/Demos/BMLwalker.html

## Chapter 3

**1** Liao, W (1990). *T'ai Chi Classics*. Shambala Publications.

**2** Van Overwalle, F and Baetens, K (2009). Understanding others' actions and goals by mirror and mentalizing systems: A meta-analysis. *Neuroimage* 2009, 15, 48 (3), 564–84 .

**3** Shapiro, S L, Carlson, L E, Astin, J A and Freedman, B (2006). Mechanisms of mindfulness. *Journal of Clinical Psychology*, 62, 373–386.

**4** Link to S Shapiro talking about the IAA model: www.youtube.com/watch?v=JjeDjhFDRfI

**5** Van Dam, N T, Sheppard, S C, Forsyth, J P and Earleywine, M (2011). Self-compassion is a better predictor than mindfulness of symptom severity and quality of life in mixed anxiety and depression. *Journal of Anxiety Disorders*, 25(1), 123–130.

Kuyken, W, Watkins, E, Holden, E, White, K, Taylor, R S, Byford, S, Evans, A, Radford, S, Teasdale, J D, and Dalgleish, T (2010). How does mindfulness-based cognitive therapy work? *Behavioural Research and Therapy*, 48, 1105–12.

**6** Haggard, P (2008). Human volition: Towards a neuroscience of will. *Nature Reviews Neuroscience*, 9 (12), 934-46.

**7** Blakemore, S J and Decety, J (2001). From the perception of action to the understanding of intention. *Nature Reviews Neuroscience*, 2, 561–567.

**8** Haggard, P (2005). Conscious intention and motor cognition. *Trends in Cognitive Sciences*, 9 (6), 290–295.

**9** Lau, H, Rogers, R, Haggard, P and Passingham, R (2004). Attention to Intention. *Science*, 303, 1208–1210.

**10** Hölzel, B K, Lazar, S W, Gard, T, Schuman-Olivier, Z, Vago, D R and Ott U (2011). How does mindfulness meditation work? Proposing mechanisms of action from a conceptual and neural perspective. *Perspectives on Psychological Science*, 6 (6), 537–559.

**11** Blakemore, S J and Decety, J (2001). From the perception of action to the understanding of intention. *Nature Reviews Neuroscience*, 2, 561–567.

**12** Anderson, D I, Campos, J J, Witherington, D C, Dahl, A, Rivera, M, He, M, Uchiyama, I, Barbu-Roth, M and Poehlman, A T (2013). The role of locomotion in psychological development. *Frontiers in Psychology*, 4, 440, 1017.

**13** Woodward, A L, Sommerville, J. A, Gerson, S, Henderson, A M E. and Buresh, J (2009). The emergence of intention attribution in infancy. *Psychology of Learning and Motivation – Advances in Research and Theory*, 187–222.

## Chapter 4

**1** Posner, M I and Rothbart, M (2007). Research on attention networks as a model for the integration of psychological science. *Annual Review of Psychology*, 58, 1–23.

**2** www.alanwallace.org/attrev.pdf provides a short summary of this book.

**3** Hölzel, B K, Ott, U, Hempel, H, Hackl, A, Wolf, K, Stark, R and Vaitl, D (2007). Differential engagement of anterior cingulate and adjacent medial frontal cortex in adept meditators and non-meditators. *Neuroscience Letters*, 421, 16–21.

**4** Hölzel et al (2007).

**5** Ekman, P (2003). Darwin, deception and facial expression. *Annals of the New York Academy of Sciences*, 1000, 205–221.

Russell, T A, Chu, E and Phillips, M L (2006). A pilot study to investigate the effectiveness of emotion recognition remediation in schizophrenia using the Micro-Expression Training Tool. *British Journal of Clinical Psychology*, 45 (4), 579–583.

**6** Doherty, R W (1997). The emotional contagion scale: A measure of individual differences. *Journal of Nonverbal Behavior*, 21 (2), 131–154.

**7** Strack, F, Martin, L L and Stepper, S (1988). Inhibiting and facilitating condition of facial expressions: A non-obtrusive test of the facial feedback hypothesis. *Journal of Personality and Social Psychology*, 54, 768–777.

**8** Brefczynski-Lewis, J A, Lutz, A, Schaefer, H S, Levinson, D B and Davidson, R J (2007). Neural correlates of attentional expertise in long-term meditation practitioners. *Proceedings of the National Academy of Science*, 104 (27), 11483–11488.

**9** Kozasa, E, Sato, J, Lacerada, S, Barreiros, M, Radvany, J, Russell, T A, Sanches, L, Mello, L and Amaro, Jr, E (2012). Meditation training increased brain efficiency in an attention task. *Neuroimage*, 59, 745–749.

## Chapter 5

**1** Smallwood, J and Schooler, J W (2014). The science of mind wandering: Empirically navigating the stream of consciousness. *Annual Review of Psychology*, 66, 31.1–31.32.

**2** Killingsworth, M A, and Gilbert, D T (2010). A wandering mind is an unhappy mind. *Science*, 330, 932.

**3** Lieberman, M (2009). The brain's braking system (and how to 'use your words' to tap into it). *Neuroleadersh Journal*, 9-14. At: http://www.scn.ucla.edu/pdf/Lieberman (InPress)Neuroleadership.pdf

**4** Lieberman, M D, Eisenberger, N I, Crockett, M J, Tom, S M, Pfeifer, J H, and Way, B M (2007). Putting feelings into words. *Psychological Science*,18, 421–428.

**5** Nummenmaa, L, Glerean, E, Hari, R and Hietanen, J K (2014). Bodily maps of emotions. *Proceedings of the National Academy of Science U.S.A.*, 111, 646–51.

**6** Batchelor, M (2007). *Let Go: A Buddhist Guide to Breaking Free of Habits*. Wisdom Publications.

7 Farb, N, Segal, Z, Mayberg, H, Bean, J, Mckeon, D, Fatima, Z and Anderson, A K (2007). Attending to the present: Mindfulness meditation reveals distinct neural modes of self-reference. *Social Cognitive and Affective Neuroscience*, 2, 313–322.

8 Craig, A D (Bud) (2009). Emotional moments across time: A possible neural basis for time perception in the anterior insula. *Philosophical Transactions of the Royal Society B: Biological Sciences*, 364 (1525), 1933–1942.

9 Nummenmaa et al (2014).

## Chapter 6

1 Van Dam, N T, Sheppard, S C, Forsyth, J P and Earleywine, M (2011). Self-compassion is a better predictor than mindfulness of symptom severity and quality of life in mixed anxiety and depression. *Journal of Anxiety Disorders*, 25 (1), 123–130.

2 Shapiro, S L, Brown, K W and Biegel, G M (2007). Teaching self-care to caregivers: Effects of mindfulness-based stress reduction on the mental health of therapists in training. *Training and Education in Professional Psychology*, 1 (2), 105–115.

3 A list of poems used in mindfulness classes: https://health.ucsd.edu/specialties/mindfulness/resources/Pages/poetry.aspx

4 Andrea Fella's teaching on AudioDharma: http://www.audiodharma.org/teacher/2/

5 Frantzis, B K (2001). *Relaxing into your Being: Breathing, Chi and Dissolving the Ego. The Water Method of Taoist Meditation (Volume 1)*. North Atlantic Books. Page 170.

6 Lutz, A, Brefczynski-Lewis, J, Johnstone, T and Davidson, R J (2008). Regulation of the neural circuitry of emotion by compassion meditation: Effects of meditative expertise. *Public Library of Science One*, 3, 1–10.

7 Luders, E, Kurth, F, Mayer, E A, Toga, A W, Narr, K L and Gaser, C (2012). The unique brain anatomy of meditation practitioners: Alterations in cortical gyrification. *Frontiers in Human Neuroscience*, 6, 1–9.

8 Allman, J M, Tetreault, N A, Hakeem, A Y, Manaye, K F, Semendeferi, K, Erwin, J M, Park, S, Virginie, G and Hof, P R (2011). The von Economo neurons in fronto-insular and anterior cingulate cortex. *Annals of the New York Academy of Sciences*, 1225, 59–71.

9 See this RSA talk for the difference in processing in the left and right hemispheres of the brain: www.ted.com/talks/iain_mcgilchrist_the_divided_brain

McGilchrist, I (2012). *The Master and His Emissary: The Divided Brain and the Making of the Western World*. Yale University Press; 2nd edition.

# Further reading and other resources

## Training with Tamara

Dr Tamara Russell's particular interest is in the embodiment of mindfulness and this lies at the heart of her two training programmes: Body In Mind Training and the Art of Mindfulness , which are offered as courses and short trainings to the general public, schools and corporations, and within the health sector.

**Body in Mind Training:** For more about BMT and how it can support your work in health, educational and corporate settings, please visit: www.drtamararussell.com

**The Art of Mindfulness:** These five-week training courses, workshops, talks, live events and other artistic projects aim to help people find their own way to living mindfully, every day. The programme explores the relationship between mindfulness, creativity and the arts, and is a creative partnership with Run Riot Projects. www.artofmindfulness.org

## A few inspiring books and websites

Blakeslee, S and Blakesell, M (2007). *The Body Has a Mind of Its Own*. Random House.

Brach, T (2007). *Radical Acceptance*. Bantam. www.tarabrach.com

Chödrön, P (2004). *Comfortable with Uncertainty*. Shambhala. www.pemachodronfoundation.org/articles/

Doidge, N (2008). *The Brain that Changes Itself*. Penguin.

Frantzis, B (2012). *Bagua and Tai Chi*. Blue Snake.

Gladwell, Malcolm (2005). *Blink*. Penguin.

Halifax, J (2008). *Being with Dying*. Shambala.

Honore, C (2005). *In Praise of Slowness*. Harper Collins. www.carlhonore.com/books/in-praise-of-slowness

Iacoboni, M (2009). *Mirroring People*. Picador.

Kahneman, D (2012). *Thinking Fast and Slow*. Penguin.

Nabben, J (2014). *Influence*. Pearson.

Tolle, E (2011). *The Power of Now*. Hodder and Stoughton. www.eckharttolletv.com

Totton. N (ed) (2005). *New Dimensions in Body Psychotherapy*. Open University Press.

Wallace, B A (2006). *The Attention Revolution*. Wisdom. www.alanwallace.org

# Index

## Author acknowledgments

Writing this book has been a real rollercoaster of moments, many of them extremely unmindful! But this process has only deepened my desire and intention to continue to embrace my mindlessness in order to develop greater mindfulness and more compassion. It's ying and yang at work. I am indebted to my family and many friends and supporters who have helped at various points in this journey, and especially to Sam Russell who has been a source of gentleness and patience. Special thanks go to my teachers, of martial arts and mindfulness, who have given me guidance and support, often in unexpected ways, but always with my development as a practitioner in mind. I know it can take years to fully understand a phrase you have heard a thousand times and thought you understood; I am grateful for their patience. I am also eternally grateful for my 'informal' teachers, those patients and clients I have met through trainings, workshops and therapeutic work. I am honoured to share a space of self-development with them; and their courage to use and experiment with mindfulness techniques has inspired me in my work and personal practice. A thank you to the many academic colleagues and friends from the Institute of Psychiatry, Psychology and Neuroscience at King's College London who have listened to me and supported me via the many formal and informal chats that have helped to shape my thinking over the years. Colleagues and friends in Barbados, Brazil and Brockwell Park have contributed greatly to my work in ways that are hard to describe – offering me space, accommodation, discussion, reflection, a place for rest, training, creativity and time to take the mini-sabbaticals needed to think and plan this work. A further massive thank you goes to Jo Childs, whose editing of the book hugely reduced the incoherent ramblings and arrived at something with more clarity and punch. Thank you also to the team at Watkins for their perseverance, patience and professionalism.

## Picture credits